MEDICINE AND MAN

Noël Poynter

PENGUIN BOOKS

Penguin Books Ltd, Harmondsworth, Middlesex, England
Penguin Books Australia Ltd, Ringwood, Victoria, Australia

—

First published in The New Thinker's Library by C. A. Watts 1971
Published in Pelican Books 1973

—

—

Made and printed in Great Britain by
Hazell Watson & Viney Ltd, Aylesbury, Bucks
Set in Monotype Bembo

Preface

THE inspiration for this little book sprang from an international symposium held in London in September 1966 under the chairmanship of Lord Cohen of Birkenhead and which I had the privilege, jointly with Dr Iago Galdston of New York, of organizing. The theme of the meeting was 'Medicine and Culture' and three days of concentrated discussion on the mutual influence existing between medicine and its cultural and social environment at various periods of history and in many different parts of the world brought together a great deal of learning and many varying viewpoints. As one of the organizers, it was my first duty to listen and learn, occasionally to question, and eventually to edit and publish the papers and discussions of the distinguished participants. Several important themes could be little more than mentioned and many questions were left unanswered.

An invitation from the publishers of THE NEW THINKER'S LIBRARY to contribute a volume to their series on this theme persuaded me to develop my own ideas and I am grateful to Mr T. M. Schuller for the continued interest which has stimulated me to write this book in the brief periods that could be spared from many other commitments. Part of Chapter 2 is based on a paper which I contributed to a symposium on 'Medicine in the City of London' organized by the Society of Apothecaries and held in St Bartholomew's Hospital. Part of Chapter 5 was used in a public lecture given in the University of Oxford in 1968, and some of Chapter 6 was expanded into a paper given at an international symposium on Medical Education in the University of California at Los Angeles and included in the volume of proceedings published by the University of California Press.

Although my own work has lain within the medical field for forty years I have never practised medicine and it is as its historian and as an observer at close quarters of many of the changes mentioned in this book that I write. Some of the views put forward here have been clarified by discussions and conversations over many years with my friend Dr Kenneth Keele, a physician of wide clinical experience and a well-known medical historian. In expressing my gratitude I must hasten to add that this acknowledgement does not imply his agreement with the arguments, criticisms or suggestions contained in the following pages. These, like any errors of fact which may have escaped my notice, are all my own. If their presentation in a volume of this well-known series provokes a wider public, as well as doctors themselves, to think about Medicine and Man in the broad perspectives of history and of the present human situation I shall rest content.

NoËL Poynter
January 1971

Contents

I

Medicine in the World Today

MEDICINE as we know it today is virtually a new creation, a product of the phenomenal scientific advances of the past century which have their own origins in the scientific revolution of the seventeenth century. Yet even in the most progressive countries it retains ideas and assumptions which go back to antiquity, and if we look around the world we find peoples among whom ancient principles and practices are still followed. The achievement of modern scientific medicine, both preventive and curative, are beyond question and are universally acknowledged. There is little doubt that eventually, unless the world returns to another dark age, it will become universally established. When people are able to choose between effective medicine and ineffective medicine the outcome is certain. The historical time-lag which has kept peoples in some parts of the world in ways of life so stable that they have become fossilized, while others have shaped new ways that have changed the whole future of man, is now being rapidly abridged. Ancient societies are being transformed in the course of a single lifetime and whole populations indoctrinated with a revolutionary zeal which provides the chief protection against the shock and breakdown which might otherwise follow the uprooting of old beliefs and institutions.

Among the peoples of European origin – and this includes those in the American continent – change, sometimes violent and disruptive, has been an important feature of their existence since the close of the Middle Ages. But the pace of change has never been so rapid as in the present century nor the test of man's powers of adaptation so severe. Hippocrates, who lived in the golden age of ancient Greece, knew that change causes illness, and it is not surprising that our age has been called 'the age of anxiety', nor that all kinds of mental illness, as well as the stress or psychosomatic diseases, are the major threat to health in western countries. These are the epidemics of our own time, following the long succession of other epidemics – plague, smallpox, tuberculosis, cholera and typhus – which have decimated the populations of earlier centuries. These have been brought under control, but tuberculosis remains a disease of poverty and overcrowding wherever these conditions persist, and especially among the impoverished and undernourished peoples of the developing countries, while occasional outbreaks of smallpox or cholera remind us how strictly the controls need to be enforced.

This is only one of the many duties of an organized public health service, which is an essential feature of government in any modern society. How effective it is depends on the skill and efficiency of its basic organization and its staff and these must depend upon the amount of money which is spent on the service. The relative expenditure *per capita* on public health in the developed and developing countries is 25:1, total world expenditure being more than £20,000 million annually. An even greater sum is spent in the United States alone on private and public financed medical care, and the annual cost of the British national health service is now close to £2,000 million. These figures reflect only part of the world effort now being directed towards the preservation of health and the cure of disease. But it is clearly not enough inasmuch as preventible and curable disease is still rampant in many parts of the world.

There is no gap in medical knowledge to remedy these conditions, only in its application, and this gap between knowledge and practice must be bridged by the sociologist, the economist and the politician. On an international scale, this is recognized by the World Health Organization at Geneva (an offshoot of the United Nations Organization), which depends for its continuing existence on the annual contributions of its member states. It has already achieved a great deal in Africa and Asia, but needs to be financed on a much more generous scale if it is to do all it could and should be doing in those areas. On a national scale, despite the increasing demand for 'fair shares' in health and welfare, few governments are able to do all that medical knowledge would enable them to do and even the most affluent country of all, the United States, has recently publicly acknowledged this gap between knowledge and performance.

A more general realization of these facts would remind us that health is not a commodity that governments can dispense as automatically as the vote and that disease is not an evil that can be abolished overnight. These are naïve assumptions which sometimes lead to an under-estimation of what is being done already. When we consider all that is involved on a world scale it will be clear that in the present century medicine and all its associated activities have become consumers of highly trained skill and manpower on a scale unparalleled in history.

The demand grows rather than diminishes, despite all that has been achieved in the last fifty years, and shows little sign of slackening in the foreseeable future. Old diseases have been mastered, but new ones take their place and the total burden of disease remains. Indeed, if we can take the annual hospital admissions in Britain as a guide to present trends it is actually increasing, for in the decade 1957–66 the statistics show a rise of over 700,000 cases, or approximately 20 per cent. On the other hand the increased effectiveness of medicine in the treatment of disease is reflected in the death rates, and especially in the infant mortality rate. In the first decade of this century 140 out of every thousand males and 114 of every thousand females died before reaching their fifth birthday; the corresponding rates are now 21 and 16. Similar dramatic falls are seen in the older age groups, the percentage improvement dropping at each stage until 65–74, when the figures are 64·8 (1901) and 53·1 (1968) for men and 53·9 (1901) and 28·0 (1968) for women. A warning sign is the fact that the figure for males in this group dropped to 51·6 in 1950 but had risen again to 53·7 a decade later. The rate of improvement is slowly declining with each decade and it seems likely that by the end of the century the rates will have become stabilized.

These statistics are sufficient to refute the idea that the phenomenal growth of medical services everywhere is a transitional phase, that the heritage of disease carried over from the wretched conditions of the masses in the nineteenth century first had to be cleared out of the way before a stable level of medical care could be reached when, with a healthier life assured for all, there might even be a reduction. More hospitals, more doctors, more research, and much more money will be demanded. How much is spent will ultimately depend on how much can be afforded rather than on needs, for these seem to be limitless.

One of the reasons for this situation is the success of medicine itself. By greatly reducing the number of infant deaths in all countries a natural check upon the rapid growth of populations has been removed. At the same time more people than ever before are surviving into their seventh and eighth decade, many of them with disabilities which require frequent medical attention. Family planning and voluntary euthanasia have more advocates than ever before, but many doctors refuse to give advice or to assist in the one, and many oppose any idea of legislation permitting the other. It could be argued that these are as essential to our social health as anything that a doctor does, but opposition, where it is not rooted in a particular religious belief, springs from traditional ethical codes in the profession which it might be dangerous to tamper with. A doctor already has, literally, power of life or death, and the relaxation of any sanctions which make it difficult for him to abuse that power should not be lightly considered. At the same time, while no member of a civilized community should suffer because of his religious beliefs, no patient and certainly no community should suffer because of the religious beliefs of some doctors or nurses. Abortion has recently been legalized in the United Kingdom and a bill for voluntary euthanasia has already been discussed in the House of Lords. More powerful government support for family planning in all countries is a certainty.

The medical profession as a whole is a conservative one. Trained to be cautious and sceptical of innovation, especially in its public utterances, it offers a restraining hand rather than an encouraging push when social reforms that concern it are under urgent discussion. Unfortunately, as the recent history of the American Medical Association leads us to believe, its advice is not always disinterested. Although the relief of suffering is a noble vocation, it has always been a desperately competitive profession, with the ways of advancement carefully guarded and narrowly routed. No other profession is so closely watchful of the actions of its members or so privately critical – and publicly silent – about any mistakes that may be made. But doctors too are human and they react to change in their status and conditions with the same shock and protest as we see elsewhere. The more devoted they are to their ancient colleges and corporations, with all their ritual and ceremony, the more strongly as a rule they react to proposed government action which may be regarded as 'interference'. But there have been, and are always some who are to be found in the van of every move for reform in health matters, among them the instigators of that very interference resented by the majority. With class barriers falling away everywhere in the world outside, the internal hierarchy of the profession is gradually giving way, but is still much more than vestigial.

Many younger doctors accept the fact that they can no longer be 'masters in their own house'. Recruits to the profession are being increasingly drawn from families that cannot afford private education and, being educated and trained entirely at public expense, with no tradition of fees being paid or received, they enter a publicly financed health service with no bias whatever towards private practice. Once fully trained a great variety of medical occupations are open to them, apart from practice with patients, and whether these are in administration, occupational medicine, teaching or research, they will become salaried employees and members of a team. Although they are by no means the best paid posts, teaching and research are a sphere where many are called and few are chosen.

It is to research that we owe the therapeutic revolution and nothing attracts like success. Medical research on the scale to which it is developed today is a modern invention. A hundred years ago it was limited to the spare-time activities of a few dozen individuals working in their private rooms (one could hardly call them laboratories) at home or in a university. Today it provides a lifetime's career for thousands of medical scientists working in specially built laboratories in universities and research institutes financed by government or the pharmaceutical industry. Research is a self-generating activity in that every step forward opens a dozen fresh paths for further exploration. Original concepts are rare and have been comparatively few in the brief history of this vast expansion, but each one (like the germ theory of disease) has led to the establishment of a new science. These are the product of chance, or intuition, and the prepared mind. Most research, much of it very fruitful in its applications, consists of the patient recording of observations and experiments designed on already established lines.

Medical research merges insensibly into scientific research which may seem of little immediate concern to the needs of medicine but from which it draws much of its sustenance. Some leaders of research now declare that there is no scientific problem which cannot be successfully elucidated if the money, time and skilled manpower are devoted to it. If we are inclined to question this somewhat proud claim we have only to recall the success of the research which has led to the landing of men on the surface of the moon. We cannot question that research must go on and that it will, sooner or later, find the solutions to the problems of which we are aware today. But recalling the present gap between knowledge and performance in medical care, it may be that more social benefit would be gained from a diversion of some part of this effort into research in the social sciences.

Despite the amount of public money spent upon research, the contribution of the pharmaceutical industry to the therapeutic revolution has been by far the more important, as a former President of the Royal College of Physicians, Lord Platt, pointed out to an august assembly of his college in a Harveian Oration. To their research scientists, many of them not medically trained, we owe the sulphonamides and the antibiotics, for penicillin only became a practical proposition after it was developed by the Pfizer Company, just as streptomycin was later developed by Merck, and all the subsequent antibiotics were discovered and developed by drug companies. 'The findings are essentially the same', said Lord Platt, 'when we look into the origins of anaesthetics, tranquillizers, vitamins, antimalarials, antihistamines, hypotensives, sex hormones, and oral contraceptives. Not one originated in a department of academic medicine or therapeutics. Even DDT, so important in preventive medicine, was discovered by Müller, working for the Geigy company.'

This is a handsome and rare tribute from one of our medical leaders to an industry at which many doctors look askance and of which governments complain because of the 'size of the drug bill' which accounts for 9 per cent of the cost of the health service. Almost the same amount is earned by the industry's exports which go to help the balance of payments. With the new drugs the sick are cured more rapidly, so that the average length of stay in hospital in 1969–70 was 10·4 days compared with 26·9 days in 1938 and 43·5 days in 1961. The industry spends lavishly on research and development; its research staff are highly qualified medical scientists, biologists and chemists, and the scale and equipping of its laboratories are superior to that of many universities. The patents which the industry is granted for its discoveries are limited to a term of years, but the price of its products is determined not by the length of this period but by the estimated speed of their obsolescence as they are ousted from current use by a new and improved drug. As research becomes more successful, the life of a new drug becomes shorter and shorter, and since research must be paid for, prices inevitably rise.

When a new compound is shown in the laboratories to arrest or cure certain diseases it is first tested on animals in case it should be found to have toxic side effects. The therapeutic revolution, which has also greatly benefited animal health, could never have been achieved without these tests, which are part of the experimental work on animals that provoke the opposition of a vociferous minority, almost entirely in Anglo-Saxon countries. Well endowed by misguided benefactors, it has a vested interest in muddled thinking and that type of sentimentality which is close to cruelty. Its activities have led to a 'Research Defence Society' and the expense of time and money which could be put to better use.

Since the thalidomide tragedy every laboratory has taken special care to ensure that any substance which has any effect at all upon embryonic development, however acceptable it may otherwise be, is at once abandoned. Once the animal tests have been successfully passed, the industry's own doctors, usually grouped together into a clinical research department, have the task of evaluating its use in human beings. The first volunteers usually come from among their own number or from their own laboratories, but every doctor either has a part-time hospital post himself, which gives him direct access to patients, or has arrangements with hospital consultants for the same purpose.

The clinical trials of new drugs are carefully planned and documented in order to be reported in a scientific paper for one of the medical journals in due course. They can last two or three years. Despite some rather ill-informed discussion on the ethical problems associated with clinical trials and complaints that patients are used as guinea-pigs, hospital patients, especially the chronic sick or those suffering with an incurable condition, are usually eager to try out a new medicine which offers the possibility of helping both themselves and others. Finally, armed with experimental records and reports of clinical trials, the company has to submit its new product for the approval of a scientific body appointed by government. In the United States it is the Food and Drug Administration; in Britain until recently the Dunlop Committee, now the Medicines Commission. There the scientific evidence is critically assessed and only after these experts are satisfied is the new drug put on the market.

No drug can ever be guaranteed to be entirely free of adverse effects to somebody. The very word 'drug' means poison and any substance which is beneficial at a correct dosage can do harm if more is taken, and any useful drug can be abused, as we know from the abuse of amphetamine among some of the younger generation. The development of 'psychotropic' or mood-inducing drugs which are non-addictive and safe promises a cure for this drug abuse as well as a new range of valuable drugs for neurosis and other forms of mental illness. This is just as well, for most doctors find it second nature to treat symptoms on empirical lines and at the same time to retain a guarded attitude towards psychiatry which is in great contrast to the fascination and enthusiasm it arouses among the non-medical. More persistent in Britain than in many other countries, this attitude probably springs from the physical segregation of the mentally sick in special hospitals which followed the nineteenth-century Lunacy Acts and the belief that little or nothing could be done for them. It is also connected with the difficulty of establishing psychiatric techniques on the same kind of scientific basis as other branches of medicine.

The mind cannot be weighed, measured, or dissected in any physical sense, but the success of the tranquillizers demonstrates that its aberrations can be repressed, if not cured, by physical means. The growing support for the idea that schizophrenia is caused by chemical changes in the brain, which could be prevented or reversed by appropriate drugs, adds to the scepticism with which certain psychological theories, especially Freudian ideas and the analytical treatments associated with them, have always been regarded by many doctors. Certainly it is by the administration of certain chemical compounds and not by the application of long psycho-analytical techniques that mental hospitals all over the world have been emptied of millions of long-stay patients, and although many have to return briefly for the treatment of acute episodes, the contribution to human health and happiness is incalculable.

Meanwhile, the number of long-stay patients in other types of hospitals increases with the ever-growing number of chronic and aged sick. The success of modern therapy is now such that the great majority of patients are either very young or very old and of these the latter represent a social rather than a medical problem. In hospital they are usually housed separately in 'geriatric' wards, but a promising development is the 'geriatric day hospital', where all efforts are made towards rehabilitation, reducing the dependence and minimizing the effects of the disability of elderly patients. By attending such a hospital for two or three days a week, patients are usually discharged after six or nine months with a much improved capacity for making the best of their remaining years.

The diseases which take increasing toll with advancing age, especially cancer and heart disease, show a steady rise in incidence but a gradual improvement in the recovery rates. Many types of cancer, if treated in good time, are completely arrested by surgery or radiotherapy, and the development of open heart surgery, with replacement of valves, veins and arteries by synthetic materials, has greatly extended the useful life of patients with serious heart disease. This type of surgery would not be possible without a good deal of physiological research dating back over the past fifty years. The kidney machines and heart-lung machines of today are the direct offspring of apparatus conceived – and sometimes made – by laboratory workers using experimental animals to elucidate scientific problems that may be far removed from those which they are now used to solve.

The development of 'spare-part surgery' has introduced new ethical problems which may require legislation to solve. The precise definition of the moment of death is much in debate at the moment because a surgeon who is waiting to transplant a particular organ or tissue wishes to remove it from the donor before it begins to deteriorate. Although spare-part banks, on the lines of blood banks, are being developed to preserve potential grafts for use, these must be in perfect condition when they are stored. The rapid development of syn-

thetic materials may make this decision less urgent than it
seems at the moment, especially if, as has happened with blood
transfusion, the number of donors fails to keep pace with
increasing demand. Even blood itself may eventually be replaced by a synthetic fluid, either wholly or partly, in emergency transfusions. Tests of possible substitutes are already
being made in the United States, where demand far outruns
supply and where the risk of serum hepatitis and other blood
infections is high. These risks are especially linked with 'free
enterprise' systems of blood transfusion, where blood is
bought and sold by middlemen who do not inquire too closely
into the medical history of their individual suppliers, who
themselves do their best to conceal an earlier illness which
might prejudice the sale of their blood. These conditions also
apply to Japan, West Germany, and Sweden, in contrast to
Britain and many other countries where the supply of blood
for transfusion is obtained almost entirely from voluntary
donors.

In this respect, as in medical care generally, the example of
Britain is more likely to be followed than the 'market system'
of the United States, not simply because it is cheaper but
because it is more efficient and less dangerous. The attitude of
the public in all countries towards medicine is ambivalent and
in the United States the love-hate relationship is everywhere
apparent. On the one hand there is a great pride in the scientific and technical achievements of modern medicine and on the
other an increasing irritation that a share of these scientific
marvels for the individual's benefit becomes more and more
costly. It is frequently said there that medical care is pricing
itself out of the market, a misleading phrase inasmuch as
medical care is not a commodity which we choose to buy or
not as we please but as we must. However plausibly economists
may present this situation it is, when stripped of all verbiage,
one in which patients are at a disadvantage in that they can

have no means of judging the true economic cost of their treatment, and if they exercise 'consumer resistance' by deferring a consultation their disease may be beyond treatment.

The increasing cost of medical care in Britain is a frequent subject of concern for successive governments, but in real terms it is not increasing as rapidly as in some other countries and as a proportion of the country's gross national product it now represents only 70–80 per cent of what is being spent in the United States. The national health service employs more than 600,000 people and staff salaries and wages represent the greatest proportion of the total cost. Since this is one sector where, even now, costs are rising by approximately 10 per cent a year, the cost of the service cannot be 'pegged' without real deterioration – that is, unless new ways are found of organizing and administering patient care in hospitals which are less expensive in time and labour than those at present used.

Although research into these problems has been going on for many years it has been generally carried out by individuals in university departments and has so far won no general agreement on the possible solutions that have been proposed. In this respect, each region is left to 'go it alone' in matching its work to its resources. Too often the answer is thought to lie in making one nurse or junior doctor do the work of three, in cutting down out-patient clinics or round-the-clock casualty departments and in closing wards, if only temporarily. That this might not be the right way to real economy seems possible if we consider the comparative costs of in-patient care in several regions, as well as those for teaching and non-teaching hospitals. These show that in the year 1969–70 the average cost in England was £55.70, an increase of 10.5 per cent over the previous year. If we look at the regional differences among the non-teaching hospitals we find the lowest weekly cost in Liverpool at £49.6 and the highest in Oxford at £60.18. If we look at the costs of each individual case, however, we find a national average of £82.51, an 8 per cent rise over the previous year, with Oxford treating each patient at the lowest cost (£69) because its staff- (and particularly its nurse-) patient ratio enabled it to do so in eight days compared with a national average of 10.4 days.

Understaffing also affects the quality of care as well as the cost-efficiency balance. Teaching hospitals, whether in London or the provinces, are usually better staffed in every department than non-teaching hospitals and the weekly cost of in-patient care in them is now running at £80.93 in London and £72.27 in the provinces. Their success rate, measured not by low-cost treatment but by mortality figures, shows some startling differences when compared with non-teaching hospitals. In the age group 45 to 54 they are 11.1 per cent of admissions for men and 7.7 per cent for women in university teaching hospitals compared with 14.9 and 14.5 respectively in other hospitals. In the age group 55 to 64 they are 16.8 and 16.4 in teaching hospitals compared with 22.4 and 22.5 in others. These statistics show what can be achieved by medical care at its best and underline the difficulty of ensuring equality of medical care, even in a national health service.

Whether they are run as private enterprise or part of a welfare state, hospitals are 'big business' that call for the kind of training, experience and skill needed in any other concern of such magnitude. Civil servants are not usually encouraged to be adventurous, the limits on their freedom of action being very clearly defined, but the National Health Service is a tremendous hotch-potch of local and national interests, of old charity and modern welfare attitudes, of old professional habits and new patient demands, all carried on without much overall knowledge of what is happening and why. Buildings themselves impose their old patterns. It is estimated that about one quarter of all in-patients need no special treatment or nursing care and should not spend long periods in bed. Better facilities for segregating really sick patients from those who are convalescing would, if more generally available, speed up recovery and allow medical and nursing staff to concentrate on those in need of their services.

The hospital is a special kind of community with its own individual character and traditions and established patterns of care which are not easy to change. When it is associated with a medical school with its own traditions orally transmitted from teacher to pupil over long periods it may be even more resistant to proposals for reorganization which may destroy its identity. When the Royal Commission on Medical Education under the chairmanship of Lord Todd published its findings in April 1968, one of the proposals which made a shudder go through the London medical schools was for the amalgamation of several of them into pairs which would create larger units more in keeping with twentieth-century developments. These schools have famous names which are known all over the world and their reputation attracts many doctors from other countries. Some are housed in obsolete eighteenth- and nineteenth-century buildings with important departments housed in basements and other inadequate premises. Foreign visitors coming from spacious and well-designed modern hospitals abroad express a sense of shock when they first encounter the reality behind the name and wonder how work of the quality produced there can be achieved in such conditions. A start has now been made by adding new blocks to old original buildings and by building an entire new hospital a few miles away from the old one. The desirability of rebuilding on original sites in the centre of a great city like London has been widely discussed and an eventual move nearer the perimeter seems inevitable.

The education which medical students receive in these schools is still essentially based on the apprentice system, with clinical teachers attempting to produce doctors in their own image. Despite attacks on the curriculum which have hardly abated over the last hundred years, it is never subjected to more than minor modifications and any kind of balanced training appropriate for the needs of the present is made difficult to achieve by the reluctance of teachers in established subjects to give up any of the time already allotted to them. Writing only ten years ago, an authority on medical education, Dr Charles Newman, pointed out that this curriculum, designed to produce the 'omnicompetent general practitioner', was still following nineteenth-century patterns rather than looking forward to the needs of the twenty-first. The Todd Report investigated and discussed this problem at length and made valuable recommendations which, if implemented, would bring about a great improvement. The Report calls for the doubling of the numbers admitted to medical schools within the next twenty years, but unless the training of these students takes more account of subjects now treated only cursorily – for example, public health and community medicine, occupational medicine, the care of the aged, and psychiatry – then old patterns will persist and even be strengthened.

Most hospitals, and most medical schools, are inward looking and tend to dismiss criticism made by outsiders, and especially the lay public, as ill-informed. As in some other public services, there is a tendency to regard them as belonging to those who staff them rather than to the people, and the end is lost sight of in their involvement with the means. Even some doctors see the dangers of a 'retreat from the patient' into laboratories, institutes and hospitals where objective study can be given to cases and diseases rather than consideration of the patient as a human being, with his family, his job and his social background, any one of which may be as important in the causation of disease as an invasive organism identified on a microscopic slide.

It is significant that many patients in India prefer to be treated in their own Ayurvedic hospitals, whatever their scientific inadequacies, rather than in that country's 'western-style' hospitals, which they regard as cold and inhuman places. Having established its own type of doctors and hospitals in its one-time colonies, Britain can now judge their effectiveness in meeting local needs. There is a valuable lesson here, not only for all who are concerned with medical aid for the developing countries but even for those who plan our medical care at home.

Some doctors – and they are usually physicians or doctors working in preventive medicine – claim that the practice of their profession gives them a special social insight which can be a valuable corrective to ultra-scientific trends and make a real contribution to medico-social problems. Practice in any large city or industrial area does indeed give many doctors an intimate experience of the seamy side of life and of the fundamental facts of existence which millions of people succeed in avoiding at first hand for the greater part of their lives. A greater emphasis on this aspect of medicine, which is likely to lead to improved methods of community medicine, is seen in an interesting development in one or two medical schools. At Guy's Hospital in London, for instance, where studies in the local ecology of their patients have been under investigation for many years, a general practice research unit has been established from which has emerged an innovation in the training of their students. This takes them outside the hospital and the school for considerable periods to work with general practitioners among their potential hospital patients. The same unit was also concerned with the planning of the new pilot scheme of medical care established in the new London suburb of Thamesmead, a completely new town with no problems of adapting or replacing old-established patterns of care. Designed on modern functional lines to give the general practitioner greater responsibility for maintaining the health of the community, as well as sufficient ancillary help to carry the increased responsibility, it should greatly ease the burden on the more expensive hospital service. Edinburgh too has a professor of general practice and in St Andrews a new research unit is taking up the work pioneered by the Peckham experiment thirty years ago and which was doing excellent work with family health until it came to an untimely end with the introduction of the National Health Service.

This side of medicine must be further encouraged if it is to earn the title of 'the humane science' which it claims to be. With its aid, positive health education, at present not nearly so effective as it should be, would be very much improved. Occasional posters and pamphlets are no substitute for the day-to-day human contact with the many opportunities for teaching by precept and practice. In these days people are likely to resent being preached at by a stranger from above, but may accept advice given tactfully by a doctor they know and regard as a friend. Although they will not be bullied into health, they can often be persuaded into abandoning unhealthy habits or practices when the reasons for doing so are explained to them. This is particularly true of mothers with children and the good work begun in the maternity clinics should be carried on by other means when the children are older.

As this side of the doctor's work is developed it brings into the medical province yet more specialist studies and journals which reflect the growing social content of medicine. Much research in the social sciences will be relevant to it and must be incorporated in the great body of existing 'literature' which covers every aspect of medical research and practice. So vast has this now become, with many thousands of specialist journals appearing regularly in all countries, that it constitutes a veritable 'information explosion'. It has long been quite impossible for any doctor to read all that is published, even in his own particular field of work, and for seventy years special indexing and abstracting journals have been appearing with the aim of ensuring that even if scientific papers and reports are not read immediately they can be found when they are needed. With the number of 'papers' (or articles) now running into millions, even these services – and the largest is financed and organized by the United States federal government – cannot keep pace and automation, or the 'machine handling of information' by computers, has now been called in to redress the balance.

This is an essential corollary to research, for by definition research should be an exploration into what is unknown, and we do not know how much we know until the information is completely organized and made accessible. When computers have succeeded in assimilating and organizing all published information the resulting synthesis will be something like the 'world brain' which H. G. Wells forecast fifty years ago and should enable many of our present anomalies to be remedied.

Indeed, the new associations of facts and ideas likely to arise from such an organized body of knowledge could itself lead to many new ideas in research and practice. New computers recently developed actually 'learn from experience' in the way that humans are supposed to do and may themselves spotlight anomalies and present new associations. Electronic machines are already performing blood counts and other routine tests almost instantaneously and so saving many skilled man-hours. They are also being developed to receive all the necessary factual information for producing a complete diagnosis, but the idea of such aids, although their introduction is inevitable, is repulsive to many physicians. They will help to solve problems of staff shortage and also to compensate for the ever-increasing need for using up-to-date scientific methods and information in clinical problems as these become more difficult.

But whatever scientific aids are provided for the doctor, his individual skill, knowledge and judgement must remain at the heart of all medical care. His difficulties do not end but may well begin with the diagnosis. The patient's family demand to know first, how serious is the patient's condition? Next they are anxious to know if the patient will recover, and then, what is the doctor doing about it? Every illness is a crisis in which the patient's individual resources, his natural resistance and personality, are challenged. Despite all that modern drugs or surgery can do, in any group of patients with similar conditions and receiving similar treatment some will recover and some will die. It is this which makes the hospital ward so different from the laboratory and it is this which necessarily makes the doctor cautious in his prognosis. He must also constantly have in mind the ancient medical maxim that whatever else he does, he must do no harm. With the powerful drugs at his disposal he must choose those which are sufficient for their purpose but which carry the least risk, for some patients respond well to a certain drug while others have adverse reactions. In certain conditions even the common aspirin may precipitate a crisis. But whatever line of treatment a doctor decides upon, he must support and reassure not only the patient but the relatives, and the good doctor does not leave this to the nurse.

When he is faced, as he is constantly, with a dying patient, sometimes referred to in emotion-saving terms as 'a terminal case', he must again act wisely and well to carry both patient and family over the period of shock. At one time, when the consolations of religion were more widely acceptable, the doctor would be aided in this task by a priest and by the understanding of relatives for whom a deathbed was not a novel experience. In a society which increasingly finds religion irrelevant to its daily life and where millions of households regard death as something which happens in hospitals and which is otherwise unmentionable, the doctor has few guidelines to help him. It is an odd feature of modern life that, just as many young husbands are encouraged to visit the labour ward of a maternity hospital to share the experience of childbirth, relatives are more and more reluctant to look upon their dead and to share another fundamental fact of life which all must experience.

These observations give some inkling of the many roles which a doctor has to fill in modern society. He must be both scientist and humanist, and while all modern trends, especially in a national service, are towards making him an 'organization man', he must retain his individual judgement if he is to do his work well as a clinician. He feels it his duty to conserve his profession's traditions, especially its ethical code, while his daily experience often tempts him to promote or support radical reforms. At times, looking around him at the whole of sick humanity, he may wish that he were a medical dictator to castigate and correct the follies and abuses which bring so many to his door. He is, in fact, neither master nor servant, but a member of a profession which has its roots in antiquity and which must continue to develop and change as an essential part of society as far in the future as we care to look.

2

Man, Disease, and History

THE history of man has often been written as the story of the rise and fall of cultures or of political empires, the struggles of rival tribes, dynasties and nations for power over others. In a broader sense, history tells of man's attempts to master his natural environment and to utilize the natural resources at his disposal for his own advancement. By the time recorded history begins, man was already a highly evolved animal, singled out from other animals by his ability to record and so to transmit his knowledge and skills, and the fruits of his own experience, to be utilized and expanded after his death. Building and the ability to make fire helped him to create an artificial climate within his own communal or individual environment. The cultivation of plants and animals provided him with food, while the dependent skills of dressing skins and weaving textiles supplied his need for clothing. Every item added to the 'necessities of life' – and this holds good for prehistoric times as well as the present age of synthetic chemicals and food additives – brings new hazards into man's environments along with its advantages. Although we have had to wait until our own time to find rivers and even seas polluted with hitherto unknown poisons, water pollution began when a stream or well of drinking-water was first contaminated by the excreta from some primitive community with a resulting outbreak of typhoid. From what we know of primitive concepts of disease, the illness and death was attributed to some maleficent spirit or sorcery, or it may have been regarded as a divine vengeance on the wrongdoings of one or more of the group.

We do not know how and when a connection between the illness and the contaminated water was first made. John Snow is credited with demonstrating this connection in 1854 during a cholera epidemic in the Soho district of London, when he advised the parish vestry to remove the handle from the pump where the afflicted families had been drawing their water. But surely such a measure of primitive hygiene must have occurred to some individual in the dim past – and perhaps he acquired a reputation as a 'medicine man' because of it. The Romans did not mix up their drinking water with the Cloaca Maxima but drew it by aqueduct from pure springs in the countryside. When Hippocrates wrote of Airs, Waters, and Places in the fourth century B.C. he knew the importance of environmental hygiene; and centuries before, in Minoan Crete, the attention to such matters is still evident in the ruins. Much must have been forgotten in the long interval, for sixteenth-century London to build its first waterworks beneath the northern arches of old London Bridge, although the Thames was already being fed by the malodorous Fleet River and other streams that were the old city's open sewers. With the river becoming more and more heavily contaminated for three centuries, the first measures of improvement only came after three great nineteenth-century epidemics of cholera, in the Public Health Act of 1875.

But there are other dangers in water, without drinking it. When it persists in undrained marshes and in stagnant ponds around dwellings, it can provide the breeding grounds for the disease-carrying mosquito. An authority on the medicine of classical antiquity has suggested that the fall of Greece was hastened by the fact that malaria became endemic in many large areas of the country. The same disease devastated the Roman Campagna for long periods and it was one of Mussolini's boasted achievements that he drained the marshes there. It was endemic in London and the Thames estuary until modern times and no remedy was known against it until Peruvian Bark (from which quinine was first extracted in 1820) was introduced into Europe by the Jesuits in the seventeenth century. The British had ample evidence of the effects of this disease in their former colonies in Africa and India. Although it was an ancient Indian medical writer, Susruta, who first implicated the mosquito nearly two thousand years ago in the spread of this disease, it was only after Ronald Ross (guided in his research by Sir Patrick Manson) demonstrated the malaria parasite inside the mosquito that adequate preventive measures were begun in the first decade of this century. At that time, some thirty million people throughout the world were still falling victim to the disease. It became one of the great humanitarian projects of the World Health Organization to eradicate malaria, the cause and means of prevention of which were so clearly established, and its advance towards this end is one of the many hopeful signs in world health which have come from that quarter. At a recent meeting of the Organization it was reported that the incidence of malaria in India has dropped by over 99 per cent in the last fifteen years, although this remains the most important single disease problem.

As in many other countries where age-old endemic diseases are at last being brought under control, in India there is a decline in infant mortality and a marked increase in population, the life expectancy being raised from 32 to 54 years, with a population growth rate of 2·5 per cent. Malaria is still the chief problem in Indonesia but a successful campaign is being pursued against smallpox with the hope of eradicating it within four years. Malaria has been eradicated from Mauritius but tuberculosis is rife there and family planning a top priority. A shortage of doctors and paramedical staff is the main concern in many countries. Although there are 8,000 new medical graduates in India every year, 80 per cent of these settle in the towns where only 20 per cent of the population live. In consequence, there is still much to be done in developing rural health services, a problem which India shares with countries like Ghana, Peru and Iraq.

Despite the social troubles which beset so many countries today, the advances made since 1945 in developing international co-operation to solve health problems, in advancing education and scientific research and in the application of new knowledge on a wide front is an important item on the credit side of the balance sheet. Many of the troubles spring from a genuine impatience with the pace of reforms and they are fed by the energies of a younger generation which, even at its most idealistic, has little or no idea of the historical background or the complexities of the problems. Nor is it always appreciated how much has already been done, and in a comparatively short time, to make solutions at least possible. Science, including medical science, is now truly international. It is in the applications of science that we find great variation, not only in the prevention of disease but also in its treatment. If we look closely at this aspect of human affairs in the world today we find conditions in one part or another which correspond to historical stages through which medical care has developed in the most advanced countries over many centuries.

There are some primitive tribes, for example some Indian tribes of South America or tribes in New Guinea, where the ideas of disease and its treatment seem to parallel closely what we know of the medicine of prehistoric man. Both India and China have well-preserved systems of medicine which are very different from the scientific medicine of the western world. The Indian system is closely related with religion and can be traced back to the ancient Vedas. The classic writings of

Charaka and Susruta, probably written nearly two thousand years ago, still provide the basis and intellectual content of practice. The Chinese system is equally ancient, its most remarkable feature being the practice of 'acupuncture' and a complicated pulse-lore aided by an extensive pharmacopoeia which contains a number of effective drugs. Although the efficacy of modern medicine is not disputed in either India or China – it is indeed scientifically taught and developed to a high research level – the ancient systems are not discarded and many millions of patients in both countries are still treated each year by the age-old methods. Pekin has its modern Institute of Indigenous Medicine and Delhi its new Centre for Ayurvedic Medicine. These are not maintained as historical curiosities but as living institutions training practitioners and carrying on research. In both countries more or less successful efforts have been made to integrate the indigenous systems with modern medicine. This has been called 'symbolic traditionalization' whereby new outlooks and methods are inculcated in a traditional guise. It is probable indeed that Indian hospitals have a far longer history than any in the west and that there was already an interchange of medical ideas and experience between Greece and India long before the time of Galen. Tradition has it that the wise king Asoka, whose reign ushered in a golden age of Indian culture, was inspired by the teachings of Buddha to establish a widespread medical service which included medical schools and hospitals, and even a hospital for animals. The rise of the great Islamic empire under Mohammed and his followers coincided with the beginning of India's decline, and its influence is still strong in modern Pakistan as well as in all the Arabic countries of the Near and Middle East. Taken over in its entirety from the Greeks, medical learning was highly regarded and embodied in a compassionate and well-organized system of medical care. All the chief cities of the Islamic world had their hospitals and medical schools and in the great hospitals at Damascus (A.D. 1160) and Cairo (A.D. 1276) free medical care was given to all, of whatever creed or nation, who came for help, with a gift of money on their discharge to help them over their convalescence. In India today there are more than 100 Ayurvedic hospitals and almost as many colleges, while native registered practitioners number more than 115,000. The great majority of the Indian people depend upon these hospitals and practitioners for much of their medical care.

The situation is much the same in China, the traditional practitioners treating most ordinary ailments while modern specialists are reserved for serious conditions requiring surgery or careful medical management.

If this seems paradoxical to Western minds, we have to remind ourselves that even in our most advanced and scientific societies there are great inequalities in the kind and amount of medical care which is available to all the population. Even in Britain, where we have a National Health Service, it is often claimed that private health insurance schemes tend to create two classes of medical care, one being inferior to the other. And if we look back over the history of medicine in Western countries there are few reasons for believing that the actual treatment of the patient, judged from its efficacy, was any better in nineteenth-century Britain than it was in second-century Rome, when Galen was bringing together all the medical ideas of his leading predecessors of the preceding five centuries, from Hippocrates on, into one coherent system. Galen knew nothing of the circulation of the blood and his anatomy was learned from animals. The well-educated physician of 1900 knew far more than Galen did of what was going on inside the body and could diagnose heart disease more accurately, but there was still little he could do for the patient.

The achievements of medicine up to that date which really

seem to have affected historical developments on a wider scale are those depending on organizational and administrative machinery. The epidemics of infectious diseases which swept through Europe periodically from Roman times on – the plague, typhus, typhoid, smallpox, cholera – left their mark on whole populations. Nobody knew why they started or why they ended and all the authorities could offer in the way of advice or help was to warn those who could to flee the affected places and for those who had to remain to shun those who were infected. Rudimentary and ineffective measures were taken to cope with terrible situations. In Elizabethan London, where plague was often an annual visitor, the dogs were killed because they were thought to be carriers. Strict regulations were enforced for cleaning the narrow streets of refuse and offal. And when a household was found to be affected it was shut up and its occupants forbidden all social intercourse. Officially such outbreaks were declared to be a punishment meted out by an offended deity and special prayers of intercession were offered in St Paul's, with special thanksgiving services when the prayers seemed to be answered and the fury of the plague was abated.

Much has been written about the Black Death which killed about a third of the population of Europe in the fourteenth century and of its economic consequences. One of its medical consequences was that from 1348–9 onwards plague became endemic in England. There were severe epidemics in London throughout the sixteenth century and many years came to be remembered as 'plague years'. The artist Holbein died in one such outbreak in 1543. Fifty years later, in 1593, when the young Shakespeare was beginning his career as poet and dramatist, many thousands died of plague in London, as they did in 1603. It is tempting to speculate on the effect which this constant threat and the daily experience of sudden death all around had upon the sensitive imagination of our greatest writer, and particularly upon the more sombre and philosophical passages of his plays. The years 1625 and 1636 were also great plague years, rivalled only by the historic and final epidemic of 1665.

Among the more lasting results of the Black Death was the modern system of quarantine. The term is derived from the Italian word *quarantena*, alluding to the forty days during which incoming vessels were detained until they were given health clearance. This began at the port of Ragusa about 1375 or earlier as a regulation for the busy maritime trade of the Venetian Republic and became of great importance in the nineteenth century when the cholera epidemics and outbreaks of yellow fever again attracted notice to the importance of such regulations.

International health regulations are today rigorously enforced, as they need to be with the growth of tourism to all parts of the world and the temporary migration of millions of people from one country to another. This control is possible only because of the accompanying growth of government machinery in all countries to the point where it is assailed as bureaucratic tyranny and an affront to the liberty of the individual. Such arguments remind us of the attacks on Edwin Chadwick, the foremost protagonist of the public health movement in England in the nineteenth century and the architect (following the lines of his master Jeremy Bentham) of our modern civil service. When *The Times* thundered that England preferred to remain dirty rather than be bullied into cleanliness by Chadwick it considered it was fighting for the liberty of the individual. The same arguments were used to oppose the Nuisances Removal Act of 1848, designed to rid the city of London of the great heaps of human ordure collected by the night-soil carts and dumped in what were called 'laystalls' as the property of individuals who carried on a trade in manure with the farmers in the countryside around

London. There is still a Laystall Street in London, but the laystalls have gone for ever, together with much else that was a permanent menace to the health of the people. But not without a struggle, and not without a sustained effort in health education and the devotion of a great many lives to its cause.

That improvements came when they did is no mere accident of history but the result of a combination of causes. First was the human environment created by the Industrial Revolution, the final relics of which are still with us although they are now rapidly dwindling in number. Intolerable conditions which were an affront to humanity and religion aroused the protests of many who shared in the wealth created in such conditions. Even some Lancashire mill owners, enlightened for their day, spent money on model dwellings for their workers and co-operated with factory inspectors in improving their workshops. Second was the rapidly increasing scientific knowledge of the infectious diseases and the manner of their spread. A bacillus or a virus knows no class distinctions and an outbreak in the hovels of the poor can swiftly attack the children in the mansions of the rich, a point that was vigorously argued by Bernard Shaw. The death from typhoid of Queen Victoria's beloved consort must have been a significant lesson to everybody. Third, it had begun to dawn upon the minds of those in authority that an industrial society depends basically on the health and strength of its workers. Even the most mechanical tasks are done better and more quickly by a healthy, adequately fed operative than by one who is ill and half-starved. With the rapidly increasing importance of international trade, commerce and finance also required a far greater number of literate workers, a consideration which could not have been overlooked in passing the Compulsory Education Act of 1870. When it was found that many children attending the new Board Schools were so sickly and undernourished that they could not profit from the lessons, a further incentive was provided for planning a centrally directed system of medical care.

Medical care is no problem if, as an individual, you can afford to pay for it when necessary without much hardship or lowering of your normal standard of living. But if a great number of people in any community are so placed that they become impoverished, and even destitute, through sickness, then any self-respecting community has to do something about it.

As a historic example of what such a community might achieve it is worth glancing at the record of the city of London. Throughout the Middle Ages London shared with the rest of the country the institutions and facilities offered by the Church for the relief of the sick poor. It was rich in monastic buildings with their infirmaries, and whatever we may think of the efficacy of medieval medicine the relations between doctor and patient were ideal for the time. For the one it was a religious duty accepted and pursued with Christian zeal, and for the other it was the acceptance of Christian charity as a religious offering which made no trespass on human dignity. Wounds and sores were dressed and healed and the patient suffering from disease was nursed and dieted with a bare minimum of drugs, simplicity and poverty enforcing an almost Hippocratic and conservative treatment which gave Nature's healing power a chance to work without too much interference.

The city of London was really a group of collectives among which the religious was the largest and the most influential. The others were the numerous craft or trade gilds into which their members were banded for mutual protection and self-discipline. Each looked after its own poor and the widows and orphans of its members. A modern parallel may be found in the workmen's medical-aid clubs, friendly societies and provident schemes that grew with the trade unions in the nineteenth century. In such 'club practice' the doctor was paid a few shillings for each member of the club and in return treated the sick whenever necessary without further charge. Apart from the gilds, to which all skilled craftsmen and artisans belonged, the pattern of medical practice before the Industrial Revolution was centred on the household, which then included a group far larger than the family. If it were a royal household, or that of some great noble, there were hundreds of retainers and servants; if it were that of a city merchant or shopkeeper, there were apprentices and domestic servants who all lived in and were treated when sick by the same doctor who treated the master and his family. As for the vagrant poor, who were drawn to the capital from places far and near, they could usually find shelter and care when they were sick and it was for just such as these that St Bartholomew's Hospital was founded in the twelfth century. From its earliest days it was supported by the voluntary and private alms of the citizens. Only after the dissolution of the monasteries by Henry VIII, when the city suddenly found itself deprived of its hospitals, was it necessary to ensure its continuance by the kind of corporate aid which only the city could offer.

It decided to accept responsibility, not only for St Bartholomew's, but also for the refounded St Thomas's, for Bethlem and Bridewell and Christ's Hospital, and in doing so it embarked on an experiment which was just as important for the sixteenth century as the National Health Service is for our own time. It was indeed the first attempt by any secular authority in Christendom to organize and maintain medical care and social assistance for its own poor. It was realized immediately that voluntary offerings would not meet the need, and the city of London became the first in Britain to exact a clearly defined and compulsory Poor Rate.

Those who could appeal for help from this source were divided into three groups: the impotent poor, including orphans and the aged, the blind, the lame and lepers; the poor by casualty, including the wounded soldier and the dangerously ill; and the 'thriftless' poor, which included the vagabond, the idler, and so on. The first two of these groups were cared for by St Bartholomew's, St Thomas's, and Christ's Hospital, then more of a hospital for sick and orphaned children than the great school which it later became. In order to provide for the third group the city persuaded the king to hand over Bridewell Palace to be converted into the first 'House of Correction' or workhouse, an institution which provided graphic material for Hogarth's penetrating art.

Fortunately, however, as with our own National Health Service, the official establishment of a comprehensive scheme did not dry up the springs of the Londoners' charity. As we learn from Jordan, the compulsory rate was supplemented by over £130,000 – then a very great sum – from individual benefactors.

By the time of Charles II the city hospitals were caring for 1,400 patients, while more than £15,000 was being spent on out-patient care. In the meantime the Elizabethan Poor Law of 1601 established the principle that pauper children must be set to work and that care should be taken of the sick and infirm. Under this law the parishes were made responsible for the treatment of the sick and injured who could not be accommodated in hospitals. The parish overseer would call in a doctor – but usually a barber-surgeon or an apothecary – and pay his fee from the parish chest. It does not seem to have been expected that the physician should give his services gratis to the poor, although as early as 1541 the Barber Surgeons' Company, just after receiving its royal charter, offered to treat up to twenty of the sick poor without fee if the city would provide a place. But physicians were not uncharitable, for three Puritan physicians gave to the poor all the fees they received on Sundays. As Sir George Clark comments: 'They do not seem to have thought of setting their Sundays apart for treating poor patients without fee.'

Even during the frequent plague years the city paid out more in medical fees than could well be afforded to the number of extra physicians who were required to take care of the infected poor. In 1641 a London physician of Huguenot descent, Dr Louis de Moulin, proposed to Parliament a corps of regular full-time salaried physicians for this plague service, as also did the College of Physicians later, but nothing came of it.

Since the early sixteenth century the population of the city had been growing by leaps and bounds. For a time the release of the monastic buildings had provided living space for the great increase in the number of families. But only for a time. During the whole of the Tudor and Stuart period there were a number of laws forbidding the overbuilding and overcrowding of tenements. The situation was exactly parallel to that which faced the public health reformers in the provincial towns of England in the nineteenth century. The great fire of 1666 gave a unique opportunity to solve this problem too, but although fine new buildings were erected, Wren's great master plan was not carried to a conclusion.

The eighteenth century saw a great new hospital movement in London inspired largely by the new merchant class. It began with the founding of the 'Infirmary for the Sick and Needy' (later the Westminster Hospital) in Petty France in 1720 and Guy's well-endowed foundation south of London Bridge in 1725. To some extent the city was already beginning to export its poorest families, with all their problems, to the outer parishes and the suburbs in order to make way for the warehouses and offices that were to serve the growing port of London and its overseas trade. But one of its most difficult problems at this time seems to have been the great number of abandoned and neglected children who were too low in the

social scale even to obtain support for their admission to
Christ's Hospital, already become a respectable school. The
connection between poverty, disease and crime, was already
dawning upon the more thoughtful observers. In his *Essay
towards the Improvement of Physick* John Bellers in 1714 lays
great stress on this and also on the economic loss to the nation
of so much wasted manpower, the real source of all our wealth,
as he rightly says, 'for without it our Country would be as
much a waste land as is America'. With the growth of the
metropolis the city's old hospitals were no longer sufficient
to serve all those in need. Bellers proposes:

That there should be built at, or near, London, Hospitals for the
Poor; if not one Hospital for every Capital Distemper; for the enter-
taining of such Poor Patients, whose Conditions may want it; And to
have Physicians and Chirurgeons suitable, to take care of the sick.

Chapter 6 of his Essay is addressed to 'The Lord-Mayor,
Aldermen and Common Council of the City of London',
whom he calls 'the Fathers, Elders, and Guardians of this rich
and populous City'. He commends them for having established a new workhouse fourteen years earlier, but begs that it
be enlarged to house

one considerable Branch of the Poor – the distressed Children
call'd the *Black Guard*, some of the most helpless parts of Humane
Nature, whose Ignorance and Necessities expose them the most
early to all manner of Immorality and Profaneness, whilst such of
them as escape are starv'd with Hunger and Cold, or some rotten or
malignant Distemper.

Bellers also proposes that the inmates of hospitals should be
given work to occupy their time and that the lands owned by
the hospitals should be worked directly for the subsistence of
the sick poor. Reckoning on the basis of 20,000 houses in the
city, the Poor Rate accounts for no more than the third part of

a farthing a day. Private alms are given lavishly in the city, but are often squandered. How much better it would be to discourage this indiscriminate charity and exact an increased Poor Rate so that the existing institutions could be enlarged and others built.

Despite his appeal to economic realism, it was private charity that set up all the voluntary hospitals in the ensuing decades – Westminster, Guy's, St George's, the London and the Middlesex Hospitals. Nevertheless, in the middle decades of the eighteenth century the number of deaths greatly exceeded the number of births and in 1741–2 reached the appalling figure of 1 in 20. Infant mortality was only a fraction below 75 per cent, and among the infants of the parish poor 80 or 90 per cent, being no less than 99 per cent among those infants who went 'on the parish' before their first birthday. The figures are those published by Jonas Hanway, the contemporary philanthropist. Thomas Coram's Foundling Hospital, which received its royal charter in 1739, at first made matters worse, if that were possible, for it became the dumping ground for all the dying and infected infants in London. The real trouble lay in the iniquitous system of 'farming out the parish poor' to a contractor for cheap labour and the parsimony of the unpaid parish overseer who was concerned only to save the rates. Viewing the contemporary scene, Dr Johnson observed that 'a decent provision for the poor is the true test of civilization'. Eventually the opinions of the civilized prevailed and in 1767 Parliament passed an Act for Parish Poor Infants which immensely improved their chances of survival. The poor called it the Act for keeping the children alive.

Other influences were also at work to provide a more humane and efficient system of medical care for the sick poor. Not least among these was the work of doctors themselves. The widespread and salutary influence of William Cadogan's

Essay on the Nursing of Children, first published in 1750, cannot be overestimated. In the same year the City Lying-in Hospital was founded and we begin to see the vast improvement in the teaching and practice of midwifery which was initiated by Dr Smellie's arrival in London from Scotland. A number of other maternity hospitals were established at this time, including Queen Charlotte's, and midwives, students and would-be specialists in obstetrics all benefited from the clinical experience they obtained in them. In discussing specialist hospitals, it is often stated that where they were established by doctors it was for their own advancement. But this is only one side of the coin, for on the other can be seen the immense benefit to the poor, not only from the more efficient and scientific treatment they received, but from actual contact with doctors, from whom they received the first principles of simple health education. It was doctors too who came most directly into contact with the sick poor in hospitals and in their own homes and who therefore knew at first hand both the actual conditions and the needs.

It was a doctor who opened the first dispensary in 1769. It was in Red Lion Square and not in the city that George Armstrong thus gave the lead to a great new movement, but many of the city's children were among the thousands whom he treated there at his own expense. In the following year John Lettsom opened the first General Dispensary in Aldersgate Street. Reviewing its progress after the first five years, Lettsom claimed that while at St Bartholomew's and St Thomas's 1 in 13 of all patients died each year (or about 600), at the Dispensary the figure was only 1 in 33. Other dispensaries followed, three or four of them within the city, and by the end of the century were proving themselves an important influence in the notable improvement of the health of the poor. Whether it was a belated proof of John Bellers's arguments of 1714, or more directly attributable to the improvements in trade and agriculture, there can be no doubt that, bad as conditions still were, they were relatively much better than fifty years earlier. Even in 1780 many of the more articulate observers were deploring what they called the 'growth of luxury' which was causing the degeneration of the people. Even the poor were drinking tea and eating wheaten bread. Dr Johnson condemned this view as nonsense. 'For Sir', he said, 'consider how small a proportion of our people luxury can reach. Luxury, so far as it reaches the poor, will do good to the race of people; it will strengthen and multiply them.'

There was in fact a widespread belief that the population was declining, but the first Census held in 1801 proved that the first fruits of the Industrial Revolution were already taking effect and that the population was on the increase throughout the country. Everywhere but in the city of London, where the expansion of trade and business was rapidly pushing the resident population off the main streets into the narrow and ill-ventilated side-streets and alleys. Where Bellers had counted 20,000 households early in the eighteenth century, by its close there were only 13,000. The figures are deceptive if we do not recall that the wealthier households had been steadily moving out of the city, west to Bloomsbury and its handsome new squares, and later southwards to Clapham. A great proportion of the 13,000 families remaining were what the College of Physicians had called 'the poorer sort', so that the City's problem of helping the sick poor was probably aggravated rather than diminished.

Heberden wrote in 1807 of the improved health of the people, claiming that cleanliness and ventilation were the chief agents in producing this reform. But there was little of either in the fever-ridden homes of the poor who congregated in the low-lying areas by the river. Infant mortality here continued as high as it had been in the eighteenth century. It is

reported that a foreigner visiting England in 1820 saw it as a
land of weeping children. In the St Giles area of London, near
New Oxford Street, in 1851, no less than 31 per cent of infants
died in their first year and 46 per cent before their second
birthday. Some of the decaying houses in that neighbourhood
were found to contain as many as 65 occupants, sometimes
four or five families in one small room, each paying three
shillings a week in rent and sleeping seven or eight in one bed.
These were houses with no water supply and no privy. So-
called 'infant nurseries', where working mothers paid as much
as five shillings a week for their children to be cared for, were
little better. And lest we should think that these must have
been isolated cases, we must recall that in Liverpool in 1837,
before the 'hungry forties' drove in more thousands of Irish
immigrants, no less than 30,000 people were found living in
7,000 dark cellars, again without water or privies. The results
in terms of health may readily be seen in the statistics of
disease and early death.

Although the plague was a thing of the past and deaths
from all kinds of 'fevers' had fallen by a third from the
average of the eighteenth century, there were still more than
2,000 a year in the city of London alone. This figure began to
decline with the opening of the London House of Recovery
(later the Fever Hospital) in 1802 and with the extra-mural
activities of its energetic committee. One of its physicians,
Dr Stanger, proposed compulsory sanitary inspection of homes
and many of the other measures taken up thirty years later by
the public health reformers.

In 1848, the city appointed its first Medical Officer of
Health, Dr John Simon, later Medical Officer to the Privy
Council. His work and experiences in the city laid the foundations and provided the model for much that was to follow,
and especially the Public Health Act of 1871. Although his
duties were not immediately concerned with the sick poor

they were everywhere involved with them. Recording this period of his career in later life he wrote:

In referring to some of the existing evils, I of course found myself face to face with immensely difficult social questions which I could not pretend to discuss; questions as to wages and poverty and pauperism; in relation to which I could only observe, as of medical common sense, that if given wages will not purchase such food and such lodgement as are necessary for health, the ratepayers who sooner or later have to doctor and perhaps bury the labourer, when starvation-disease or filth-disease has laid him low, are in effect paying the too late arrears of wages which might have hindered the suffering and the sorrow.

Shaw himself never put this argument more succinctly.

By this time the Elizabethan Poor Law had given way to the New Poor Law of 1834, which emphasized the 'deterrent' principle by concentrating relief in the workhouses but which made no official provision at all for the sick poor. This grave oversight was gradually remedied by the Poor Law Commissioners (later the Poor Law Board), but only with great difficulty and after a tragic wastage of human lives. What is quite certain is that Victorians were not blind to the prevailing evils. It was after all Victorians who agitated for better conditions and eventually were rewarded by the Metropolitan Poor Act of 1867 and the later Public Health Acts. The former was the work of a conservative government and is worthy of closer historical study. It was in fact a most revolutionary Act, yet it went full circle and returned to the first principles of the Elizabethan committee which had classified the indigent poor. Once more the sick, the lunatic, the children and the able-bodied, were to be cared for, not in a common workhouse, but in separate institutions, just as the city of London had decided in the reign of Edward VI. Only this time the unit was to be larger and all the unions of the metropolis, now spread far beyond the city, were to be joined for the purpose of establishing and maintaining institutions for the free medical care of the sick poor. They were to be governed by a central authority, the Metropolitan Asylums Board, and financed by a Metropolitan Common Poor Fund. It was a pattern that endured until the Local Government Act of 1929, when the Board's hospitals were taken over by the London County Council. The institutions taken over at that time numbered more than a hundred, with a grand total of more than 75,000 beds, by far the largest such complex for which any local authority in the world was responsible. Less than twenty years later the metropolitan model was enlarged to cover the whole country through the National Health Service.

Much has had to be omitted from this brief account of medical care in the city of London. As the metropolis of a great trading and manufacturing nation it serves as an appropriate case-study. The city began with the right ideas – the ideas to which we had to return in the last century – but it was overtaken by the speed of its own growth and by its own fatal attraction for the poor and needy who saw there a hope of better things. Individual charity was poured out by private citizens in an effort to relieve distress that was beyond the means of the city's own institutions. But the problem was too great for that and had to await State intervention for its proper solution, first in 1867, then again in 1929, and finally in 1948.

On each occasion there have been those who tried to stem the tide of history and those who travelled with it. In the days of Queen Victoria there was one notorious Dr Chalmers who believed that 'charitable gifts from the hands of district visitors could and should take the place of the Poor Law, and that the virtue of humanity ought never to have been legalized, but left to the spontaneous working of man's own willing and compassionate nature'.

On the other side was Lord Hobhouse, whose view was forcibly expressed in his paper on Charitable Foundations in

1868, in which he condemned the motives of their founders as 'love of power, ostentation, and vanity'; while Gladstone in a Budget speech of 1863 proposed to tax endowed charities as he considered them to be of very doubtful value. Hospitals alone among the charities were still regarded as worthy objects of charity, and continued to be so regarded until 1948. After an initial setback when the old voluntary hospitals were taken over by the State, the springs of charity are flowing still, but more strongly now towards medical research, the fruits of which will probably help rich and poor alike.

If we can learn anything at all from history then the message to be found in this brief narrative is surely that the National Health Service, produced after such difficult and prolonged labour and the subject since 1948 of perennial controversy, was not in fact a revolutionary scheme, but the natural consequence of all that had been pointing the way for it during the preceding 400 years. Much of its so-called 'free' element can be found in full measure in older and more compassionate societies unclouded by the criticism, or even anger, which this arouses in the rugged individualist of today. In fact, it is he, and not the compassionate society which may be seen as the 'sport' or freak in the course of natural development, perhaps a mutation encouraged by the hectic competitive spirit of the Industrial Revolution. As for the N.H.S. family doctor, he is the heir of the 'panel doctor', who from 1911 on was treating under a State insurance scheme only the breadwinner in the family. And the panel doctor is the heir of the 'club doctor' and the workhouse doctor, each of whom treated a great number of people for a set annual fee, while both are the heirs of the parish doctor who treated his neighbours – at least the poor who made up the majority – for less than ten pounds a year.

3

Medicine and Religion

ONLY a year or so before the outbreak of the Second World War a French writer committed to print the statement that 'Science would make us gods before we are worthy to be men'. In his Reith lectures in 1969 Dr Edmund Leach declared that 'Men have become like gods. Isn't it about time that we understood our divinity?' The thirty years between these two utterances have been remarkable for calculated destruction, massacre and sheer human misery on a scale hitherto unknown to history. Whether we attribute this to temporary mass insanity, original sin or to the temporary triumph of evil in the world, this juxtaposition of opinions offers food for thought to both the psychiatrist and the orthodox religious of all creeds. The definition of a 'god' has been the subject of innumerable theological discourses and any attempt at providing one here would take us too far from our present purpose. It is enough to say that most Christians would agree that it is the merciful aspect rather than the omnipotent which the doctor keeps before him – a god of love rather than of vengeance. The scientific positivism which has transformed medicine – to the point where some foresee a time when diseases may be entirely prevented or successfully treated – has also made it less necessary than ever before for the doctor to seek or recommend metaphysical consolation for the suffering which is beyond his powers of treatment. At a time when controversy centres upon ethical problems such as family planning, abortion, organ transplants, euthanasia and so on, problems of which we shall have more to say in a later chapter, medicine and the Church seem to be in opposite camps. Some even ask themselves what such problems have to do with religion at all. The population explosion which is worrying so many people with a real concern for the future welfare of mankind seems likely to transfer them from the ethical field to an internationally agreed political programme. Until politicians catch up with the facts of life, the responsibility for deciding these matters of life and death rests with the doctors.

The dialogue between religion and medicine has been going on for a long time. Long before medicine became an important part of Greek philosophy (which also embraced the biological and physical sciences) it was deeply rooted in religion. In ancient Egypt, the priests were physicians, and from Egypt the early Greeks borrowed the idea of so-called 'incubation'. The equivalent of the modern hospital was the temple of healing, to which the sick came to be cured. At Epidauros can still be seen the ruins of the great temple of Asklepios, the founder of Greek medicine who was made a god, and close by are the buildings erected to house the thousands of sick people who flocked to it. The cure began with a process of spiritual and physical purification, after which the patients were led to one of several galleries near the temple and told to sleep. In their dreams the god himself appeared to them, either curing their condition immediately or instructing them what they were to do to be cured. On their departure the grateful patients left a permanent token of their cure in the form of a terra cotta or even marble representation of the affected organ or part of the body, while details of the cure itself were often inscribed on tablets which have survived into our own time.

Anybody who knows well the cathedrals of Italy, Spain and France cannot help being reminded of certain chapels in them dedicated to one or other of the 'healing saints' to which sufferers have come to pray for aid, leaving behind them a miscellany of souvenirs of their former condition. And of course there is Lourdes.

Ancient temples and medieval shrines also serve to remind us of two facts: first, that throughout history there have always been diseases which no doctor could cure; and second, that the human mind has within itself, given the right conditions, the power to heal the body. Especially does this apply to mental illness and the so-called psychosomatic disorders. The good doctor not only acknowledges this but uses his knowledge daily in his practice. He would much rather see the cancer patient for whom he can do no more seeking consolation and support in religion than in dangerous and useless quack remedies.

The rise of Greek science did nothing to oust the cure by incubation. The rational and naturalistic approach of Hippocrates to the phenomena of disease developed side by side with the religious approach and was eventually brought into a complete system of medicine by Galen in the second century A.D., at the very time when the new religion of Christianity was winning followers in the Roman world. The healing miracles of Christ epitomized much of its appeal for the sick and the suffering. When the Church of Christ became a great temporal power, controlling all learning, it had to incorporate medicine as part of that learning. Although not himself a Christian, Galen was the pagan writer whose account of the workings of the human body and its disorders had in it little that was offensive to Christian teaching. He saw in the wonders of bodily structure a miracle of design, with every part expressing the divine purpose, a feature which also made it acceptable to the devout followers of Islam in the eighth century, so that his writings became the basis of the work of their greatest physician, Avicenna, often called the 'Arabic Galen'.

Muslims, no more than Christians, were allowed to dissect

the human body, which had to be preserved intact for religious reasons, so that Galen's own interpretation of his studies on animals had to be accepted almost as an article of faith, an act which was in complete harmony with a society where religion permeated every aspect of life. St Augustine, following the neo-Platonists, insisted that the way to knowledge was by divine revelation and this was official doctrine until St Thomas Aquinas in the thirteenth century revived the intellectual rationalism of Aristotle in his celebrated *Summa*, a systematic exposition of the officially accepted knowledge of his time.

In the meantime, on the more practical level of everyday life, the concentration of education within the Church and the rise of the monastic orders resulted in a situation where the majority of those practising medicine were themselves churchmen. Particularly skilled and able practitioners were often called upon to travel great distances for the treatment of some high churchman or noble and to remain for long periods away from their monastery. The effect of this kind of life upon their keeping of their monastic vows was only too apparent so that eventually, in the twelfth and early thirteenth centuries, new regulations were introduced forbidding clerics (with certain conditional exceptions) to study medicine or surgery or, if they were already trained to do so, to be absent from their monastic house on medical affairs for more than two months. It is important to mention this ban, for it has been misunderstood and elaborated (by an eighteenth-century fiction) into the famous phrase *Ecclesia abhorret a sanguine* which has misled many historians and given rise to the belief that the Church was responsible for the division of medicine from surgery.

The rise of the universities at this time helped to provide more and better trained doctors, especially in those universities such as Bologna, Padua and Montpellier, where medicine was highly regarded. It has been claimed, although this claim is not generally accepted, that it was in Padua in the fifteenth century that there was developed that objective and independent method of scientific investigation to which modern medicine owes so much, and that this came about because Padua enjoyed the support and protection of the Venetian Republic and was not answerable to the Papacy. It is true at any rate that Padua was the university of Vesalius, whose objective studies of the human body overthrew Galenic authority, of Copernicus, who transformed men's view of the universe, and of Galileo, who was attacked by the Church for his revolutionary enunciation of natural laws.

Other medieval foundations of more immediate concern to the practice of medicine were the hospitals. When the first Christian emperor of Rome, Constantine, closed all the pagan healing temples in A.D. 335, he was persuaded to encourage Christian foundations to take their place. The oldest Christian hospital, of which St Gregory has left a description, was founded at Caesarea in Cappadocia in A.D. 369 by St Basil, an example which was followed rapidly throughout the eastern empire. The Hôtel Dieu in Paris, the oldest surviving hospital in western Europe, was founded about A.D. 650 by St Landry, bishop of Paris during the reign of the Merovingian king Clovis II. The title is a French rendering of the Latin *Domus Dei*, which stresses the religious character of the foundation and some idea of what it was like may be gained by a visit to St Mary's at Chichester, an Hôtel Dieu which has survived from Anglo-Norman times and is now an almshouse. It is important to remember that it was not only a home for the sick, but also for the homeless and the wayfarer as well as for a few individuals who wished to retire from the world. Medical care was simple and compassionate, the diet spare but wholesome, while the presence of the altar in their midst reminded the occupants of their religious duties and the fact that healing was a spiritual as well as a physical act. Our own oldest hospital, St Bartholomew's, founded as part of an Augustinian priory in A.D. 1123, must have been very similar, although its rebuilding at the beginning of the eighteenth century has obscured the resemblance.

The existence of such a retreat could benefit only a minority of the sick. For the majority, such treatment as was available – and it was briefly limited to purging, blood-letting and 'diet-drinks' – was given at home. More serious ailments might be the subject of prayer or of special intercession at one of the healing shrines which abounded throughout Europe. When the Reformation came some of the intellectual protest against the abuse of religion and the growth of superstition spilled over into medical practices too, so that the Swiss physician known as Paracelsus openly defied the classical medical authorities enshrined in the universities and burned their books in the market place. This man, who has been called the 'Luther of Medicine', was as devoutly religious as Luther. He believed that the presence of God was manifest throughout all nature, including disease; that where there was disease God also provided the cure in the medicinal herbs that grew in the vicinity, their use being indicated by their outward characteristics, an idea that gave rise to a crop of national and local 'herbals', the books on medicinal plants which are the forerunners of the official pharmacopoeias. In England the idea was taken up by Timothy Bright and Culpeper and survives in the little handbooks and catalogues of the modern herbalist. This belief that God places the remedy close to the disease was mentioned again towards the end of the last century when it was found that acetylsalicylic acid, extracted from the willow which grows in damp places, was useful for rheumatism, commonly believed to be caused by living in such areas.

But if some found in this association further reason to praise the wisdom and beneficence of the Almighty, others questioned the reasons for the creation of diseases in the first place. Despite the fact that medicine was traditionally regarded as a vocation, implying a religious motivation, doctors had always been notable doubters and Chaucer reminds us that in the earlier centuries when the Church was supreme the doctor was often suspected of atheism. At that time, and for long afterwards, medicine was the only formal study by which one could acquire some knowledge of the subjects that are today included under the term 'science'. Many simple experiments and demonstrations that are now carried out daily in the classroom were then regarded as magic. The chemist was still the alchemist, and the doctor was primarily concerned with his search for the elixir of life that was to cure all diseases, if only incidentally with his search for gold. Nevertheless, the doctor's mental reservations did not stand in the way of his outward conformity, for he was a prominent figure in society. He officially subscribed to the view of the theologians that disease was sent as a punishment from God, for he could not suggest any more precise causation, and when a great plague struck at a whole people he was present at the service of intercession as well as at the thanksgiving service when the danger was seen to be over.

Living as we do in an activist society, where every kind of social ill provokes shouts of protest and demands for the government to *do* something about it, we find it hard to appreciate the extent of the fatalism with which our forefathers faced all the hazards of their daily life. That this fatalism had a great deal to do with religious belief and with the orthodox view of the after-life is apparent in the teachings of the Church throughout the ages. One of the most important and far-reaching of the social reforms which revolutionized the life of the people in the nineteenth century was the establishment of a modern system of public health, first in Britain, where the evils associated with the Industrial Revolution first became apparent, and later in other countries. Much has been written about the leader of this movement, Edwin Chadwick, and the 'sanitary idea':

What, it may be asked, was Chadwick's 'sanitary idea', the root-principle which inspired his life-work? It was, according to Richardson, 'that man could, by getting at first principles, and by aiming at causes which affect health, mould life altogether into its natural cast, and beat what had hitherto been accepted as fate by getting behind fate itself, and suppressing the forces which led up to it at their prime source.' To this end, direct investigation on the spot into the removal of the preventable antecedents of disease and crime claimed his attention. . . . He dwelt on unity of purpose in the prevention of evil.

Although this is true as far as it goes, it does not go far enough. If we search into the intellectual origins of this movement we find that it began with a change of religious belief by a man who became the eloquent evangelist of sanitary reform. This was Dr Southwood Smith, Chadwick's medical colleague in the first General Board of Health, and the man who first expounded the sanitary idea to Chadwick when the latter was a young lawyer. Smith had been brought up and educated to become a Calvinist minister. At the age of 19, while still a student at the Bristol Baptist Academy in 1807, he revolted against the Calvinist teaching that the majority of mankind were predestined to eternal damnation and that only a small group of the elect were to be saved. He turned to Unitarianism and became a minister in its church in Edinburgh at the same time as he studied for a medical degree. His evening sermons attracted great crowds and in them he argued that in the light of the Divine Wisdom the only purpose of punishment could be redemption, not revenge. The work of redemption could be begun in this life and the implications of what he called the doctrine of 'universal restitution' were that 'What *can* be improved *must* be improved and *will* be improved until man in society reflects the benevolent purpose of the Almighty.'

His first book, entitled *Illustrations of the Divine Government*, was based on these sermons and was published in 1816, when Chadwick was still a boy. It earned the praise of both Byron and Wordsworth. In the preface to the third edition, published in 1822, Smith wrote,

I have considered, separately and in detail, the several classes of evil, namely, natural and moral evil, and the evils which have hitherto been found inseparable from the social state, namely poverty, dependence, and servitude. . . . There is a closer connexion than there might at first sight seem between these subjects and those (that is, medicine and sanitary reform) which now much more exclusively occupy my attention: the real end of both is the same; for the object of each alike is to extend the knowledge, to mitigate the suffering and to increase the happiness of mankind; and without doubt that is the great business of life.

He argues against views and theories which 'tend to degrade man in the estimation of man and represent him as too cheap. This low estimation of the value of a human being', he writes, 'this contempt of human nature, is fatal to human improvement and is at the foundation of the enormous errors of statesmen and the gigantic crimes of warriors; they could not squander life and violate happiness as they do, did they judge man as he is.'

It is significant that before Southwood Smith began his life-work the definition of a 'humanitarian' was 'one who denies the divinity of Christ', that is a Unitarian, a follower of the old Arian heresy which asserts that Jesus Christ was not God, but a human being. Before he had completed it the term was already being used widely to mean one who found 'the great business of life' in mitigating the sufferings and increasing the happiness of mankind.

The struggle against poverty and disease found many

doctors devoting their lives to this 'great business'. They, more than other men, saw the enemy at close quarters and had the education and the ability to tell of what they saw. Many, like Smith himself, were urged on by their enlightened religious beliefs, and they found strong allies. Foremost among these was Florence Nightingale, the founder of modern nursing, who never minced her words in flaying 'the enormous errors of statesmen' and demonstrating in action the value of human life. She too found an unfailing spring of energy in her religious belief which, if not entirely orthodox, was lasting and profound.

Florence Nightingale was born in 1820, only a year before Mary Baker Eddy, and both died in 1910. No greater contrast could be found in any two historical figures than is apparent in the characters and achievements of these two women. Mrs Eddy was the founder of the system of faith healing known as Christian Science. It arose at a time when many strange quasi-religious cults and sects flourished in the United States and it drew its inspiration from a New England watchmaker named Quimby. He began by dabbling in mesmerism and so-called magnetic cures, a part of 'fringe medicine' which had amused and intrigued fashionable society in Europe for several decades after it was begun – and discredited – in Vienna and Paris by the German doctor, Franz Mesmer. After a time Quimby found that the elaborate ritual laid down by Mesmer was quite unnecessary, the cures being effected by simple hypnosis and suggestion, therapeutic aids that were by no means unknown to orthodox doctors but which still awaited the widespread use now seen in psychiatric practice. After a successful 'treatment' by Quimby, Mrs Eddy became his disciple and the leader of the new cult after Quimby's death in 1866. It was she who was responsible for developing it to the level of a new religious sect, largely through her book *Science and Health with Key to the Scriptures* (1875), founding the first of her numerous churches in Boston. It drew its strength from the fact that neurosis is a common ailment in the cure of which faith healing can be most effective.

The mission of the Christian Church from the beginning had been to heal the sick as well as to preach Christianity and, even when many of the old rituals associated with therapy were abandoned at the time of the Reformation, the powerful agency of prayer was recognized and widely used, as may be seen from the English Prayer Book. To this extent, there was nothing new in 'Christian Science' and had this been its sole aim it would hardly have incurred the hostility of orthodox medicine. This hostility was not a reaction to prayer and faith healing but to the teaching that sickness did not exist except as human error, and that consequently there was no need for doctors. This teaching has led to a refusal on the part of Christian Scientists to accept the help of doctors, even in acute emergencies, and sometimes on behalf of children too young to decide for themselves. Vaccination, blood transfusion and emergency surgery have saved the lives of millions, but the overwhelming weight of evidence has no effect on those who deny their validity on religious grounds.

Christian Science, along with some other modern sects which share their views on orthodox medicine, are outside the main stream of historical development in which religion (and not only the Christian religion) is seen to be closely concerned with the profession and practice of medicine. It is true that in modern scientific medicine it may seem to be acceptable only at the delivery point, as it were, where the doctor faces a patient and his individual problems, whether he is in a hospital ward or at home. But it must be remembered that in many areas of the world, former colonies of the European nations, the first effective medical care on modern lines was made available to the people through the work of Christian missions. These may not enjoy the popular support they once

had, but the life and work of medical missionaries such as
Dr Albert Schweitzer leave no doubt of their sincerity and
dedication. The same spirit animates many who work among
the underprivileged nearer home where the doctor and the
priest are still the only public figures who are accorded some
measure of respect.

Just as the work of the doctor is often inextricably en-
tangled with problems of social welfare, so too is that of the
minister of religion. There is in Britain an Institute of Religion
and Medicine which counts the Archbishop of Canterbury
and Sir Arthur Porritt among its past presidents. Reporting
the work of its field and study groups throughout the country
it declares its aims to be to help the sick and to promote the
health of the community. 'It also seeks to foster inter-profes-
sional co-operation so as to minimize the anxieties and dissatisfactions experienced by its members in their work with
individuals and in their contact with each other. It also tries to
influence medical and theological teaching so that modern
concepts of personality, relationship, and communication are
fully used in the healing process.'

Its basic assumptions are that:

As health is a function of the total relationship between the individual and his environment it must involve his physical, mental and
spiritual well-being.

So the promotion of health and the healing of the sick is not only
the particular concern of doctors, it is something which also concerns
members of associated therapeutic professions and religious leaders.

Currently in our society there is both a fragmentation of endeavour
and a failure of communication and understanding between the
various professions who should rightfully be concerned about this
vital problem.

Equally the community in general and its leaders in particular need
to consider how society can best be structured to heal the sick and
promote the well-being of its members.

While doctors and theologians attempt to diagnose and prescribe for the ills of modern society, other forces tend to aggravate them before they can be treated. The so-called permissive society, a manifest sign of the all-pervading influence of Freudian theories, has abandoned many of the moral sanctions which once buttressed orthodox religion and a disciplined community life. The church is no longer the central figure of that life as it was for centuries, as the mosque still is for Muslims and the temple for Hindus or Buddhists. Whereas attendance at a church service was once the chief community activity of millions, it may now be given a lower order of priority, or dropped altogether, in favour of a football match or a political demonstration. It has been argued that the decline of religious observance has left many individuals with little or no community contact, and that this is one of the factors in the notable increase of mental illness. This may well be true, especially among the elderly. Despite the religious injunction to 'honour thy father and thy mother', one of a doctor's problems today is how to persuade the sons or daughters of ailing and aged parents to take them back into their home once they have spent a period in hospital. How frequently he fails to do so may be seen in the crowded 'geriatric wards' of any local hospital. With a rapidly ageing population, this break-up of family life into smaller and smaller units presents a problem of community health which is yet to be fully appreciated.

At the other end of the scale are the hundreds of thousands of adolescents who have broken away from their families and actively repudiate the moral standards and way of life of their parents. The 'drop-outs' and the drug addicts present an ever-increasing medical as well as social problem which legislation alone cannot solve. The latest report of the Chief Medical Officer of Health informs us that in the last year there were no less than 1,232 children born to unmarried girls under the age of sixteen and another 1,213 abortions in the same age-group, representing a demand on medical and welfare resources which are already stretched to capacity. The Church has always been the guardian of morals and the traditional disciplinary agent has been the concept of sin and guilt. At the present time even the strongest and most highly organized of the Christian churches, the Roman Catholic Church, seems to be fighting a rearguard action against growing demands for a revision of its views on such matters as contraception, abortion and euthanasia, all matters with which doctors are closely concerned. A century ago such demands and the ensuing discussions and debates would have been known to comparatively few. Now, with universal education and the existence of powerful means of world-wide communication in the form of television, the debates themselves can be heard and seen by millions, a fact which cannot fail to harden the attitudes of the chief participants, leading to the over-simplification of complex problems and to their popular presentation in terms of black and white.

Not all churchmen are inflexible in their approach to the great moral problems of the time. Not all doctors see the Church as an obscurantist and reactionary body standing in the way of a social solution of many medical problems. In his professional capacity, however, a doctor's chief concern is with the physical and mental well-being of his patients. In his practice he is confronted daily by situations which may exercise his conscience and challenge his religious belief. If he works in a typical urban and industrial area, he will probably find that only a small minority of his patients are practising Christians and that the rest are not prepared to accept his guidance on what is right or wrong for them. Many find that the application of readily available scientific means is more effective in mitigating human suffering than religious or moral exhortation. Resigned or disillusioned he may become, but all his training prevents him from adopting a purely negative or passive attitude.

Many question the relevance of religion to any of these problems. Moral standards are never absolute. They are different in different societies and have varied greatly in the same society at different historic periods. It was once considered moral to whip lunatics, or to keep them chained and naked in dark cellars. It was once considered moral to hang the mother of starving children for stealing a loaf of bread. The sanctions needed – or thought to be needed – to safeguard any community against potential transgressors of the rules which preserve it are constantly changing, so there is no reason to suppose that society will suddenly cease to adapt itself to changing customs and ways of life. Nor are religious outlooks fixed forever in their present form, as we are reminded by some of the cardinals in the Roman Catholic Church, for that too has survived by adaptation.

The Church has always been very much concerned with the moment of birth and the moment of death, the two occasions in life when doctors are most likely to be present. In the days when a high proportion of new-born infants died in their first month of life the Church placed great stress on infant baptism, for the soul of the child who was not baptized could never go to heaven but would linger forever in limbo. It was therefore important that the doctor should appreciate the urgency of these religious ceremonies and make sure that any infant whose life was uncertain should be baptized immediately, if necessary in the birth chamber. When theologians began to debate the precise point in a pregnancy at which the soul enters the body, their religious solicitude extended to the ante-natal state and in the seventeenth and eighteenth centuries led to the baptism of the child while it was still in the womb and some of the instruments devised for this purpose have survived.

It is held to be equally important that at life's end the dying person should have the opportunity to confess his sins and to make an act of contrition and receive absolution. It is for this reason that chaplains of various religions and sects are often to be found in hospitals, not merely for visiting the sick, where they may or may not bring comfort, but to perform the last rites for the dying members of their own faith. It is here that those who propose voluntary euthanasia find their greatest obstacles, for the religious insist, quite rightly according to their beliefs, that whatever the physical condition of a patient, as long as a spark of life persists there is still time for the soul to make its peace with God. That the prolongation of life as long as possible is also the traditional ethical duty of the doctor probably has its basis in the same consideration. The supporters of euthanasia do not dispute the rightness of this action for religious believers but they do point out that it is often imposed upon non-believers who sincerely believe that there is no after-life and who wish to spare prolonged distress to their families and to depart this life with dignity.

This problem is also closely linked with transplant surgery, where a surgeon has to remove tissues or organs with all possible speed in order that the life of another may be prolonged. The possibility that death may be hastened for this purpose, in cases where there is no hope of survival, has sparked off debates on the medical and legal definition of the precise moment of death. Since modern physiology has made it possible, with the aid of machines, to extend the life of patients who, without their use, would certainly die, the question arises, Who switches off the machine? And when? Some patients with severe brain damage are kept 'alive' in this way, in coma, for months or even years, being given constant monitoring and specialist care. It has been known in such circumstances for nurses and patients who know of it, their pity aroused, to call such a procedure 'inhuman' and to ask why it is continued. But it is a strange quirk of human nature that makes these same compassionate observers, when the switch is eventually pulled, turn their faces away, at least for a time, from the doctor who was responsible for the decision. This reaction throws light on the human difficulties surrounding the whole subject of euthanasia. The doctor should not be made a scapegoat. The religious are taught to pray for an easy death, but if prayers are not answered they are reluctant to allow any human agency to bring about what God has not granted.

For every extreme case, such as that mentioned above, there are thousands where, with survival impossible, death is postponed for weeks or even months with the aid of modern drugs and scientific techniques. The patient, especially if old and weary, is not always grateful, but relatives are satisfied that 'everything possible has been done'. Doctors have to use the means available to them, if for no other reason, lest they should be charged with negligence. The irony of the situation lies in the fact that these techniques have been developed from laboratory experiments on animals, including vivisection. The religious motives which demand that every means should be employed to prolong life were also responsible for a flourishing anti-vivisection movement which is, and has always been, at its strongest in Britain and which has propagated an image of the researcher using animals as a sadistic and cruel monster. The attitudes are not consistent, but it is not only the religious, but our whole society which needs to think seriously about this problem and to discuss possible solutions which meet the emotional, the religious and moral difficulties. A former editor of the *Lancet*, Sir Theodore Fox, was outspoken on this issue when he said, 'But unhappily there are also patients and relatives whom this rule (i.e. for the prolongation of life) condemns to needless suffering. . . . I cannot think myself that human societies should compel a dying citizen to suffer for the sake of others; or if they do so compel, the medical profession should not abet them.'

Apart from a slight reference to Greece and Rome, most of this chapter has been concerned with the relations between medicine and the Christian religion, but some reference must be made to the religion which has exerted such an over-whelming moral and ethical influence on Christian society, that is, Judaism. That 'cleanliness is next to Godliness' has become proverbial, but it springs from Talmudic teaching and Jewish laws of hygiene go back for more than three thousand years. The Old Testament is full of sound advice for social and personal hygiene and strict rules guard the health of the orthodox. Ritual bathing and the careful washing of hands after any action that might contaminate them, especi-ally before meals, prevent much infection. The classification of animals used for food into 'clean' and 'unclean' leads to the avoidance of pork and shell-fish, which are among the com-monest causes of food poisoning. The ritual slaughter of food animals is painless and immediate and the draining of all blood greatly increases the keeping properties of the meat, especially in a hot climate. Particular stress is put upon sex hygiene, with circumcision and careful rules about menstrua-tion as a central feature, while the forbidding of consanguin-eous and incestuous unions is justified by what we now know of genetics.

With preventive medicine and public health so closely integrated into religious belief it is no coincidence that the Jews have throughout history provided many famous doctors and medical teachers. One of these, Moses Maimonides (1135–1204) was both Rabbi and physician and some of his own rules for the maintenance of health are incorporated into the Jewish code of law.

Another religion with the same fastidious regard for the

rules of hygiene is Hinduism. A strict code of personal hygiene and sanitary practice is embodied in the laws of Manu, dating from the year A.D. 200. These require every practising Hindu to bath every morning and to clean his teeth with a twig from a certain tree which is not used more than once. Shoes must be discarded on entering a house and clean clothes must be worn for the preparation of food, in the cooking and eating of which scrupulous attention must be paid to cleanliness. Alcohol is forbidden and water is the common drink, while regular ritual fasts and periods of abstinence from the eating of meat prevent obesity and the diseases that follow in its train.

But India also has an indigenous system of medicine, Ayurveda, which is complete in every respect and which has its roots in antiquity. Ayurveda comprises all the body of medical knowledge contained in the sacred books of the east, some of which go back to periods before Hippocrates. Indeed, some scholars think that the influence of ancient Indian medicine and science can be traced in the writings of the ancient Greeks. The two ancient *Samhitas* by Charaka and Susruta crystallize that medical and surgical knowledge in texts which are still printed and used today. Resting largely on a vast botanical lore and the use of many kinds of medicinal plants to cure various disorders, Ayurvedic medicine, and indeed the whole Indian way of life with its social harmony and spiritual aspirations, is permeated with religion and it is perhaps not mere coincidence that mental illness is less of a medical problem in India than in any western countries.

In India, as in many other parts of Asia and Africa, the development of modern scientific medicine is often hindered by religious rules and beliefs the importance of which is not always appreciated by western advisers. It is not sufficient for these to be trusted medical specialists if the developing integration between ancient beliefs and modern science is to be pursued. They must be assisted by men and women of wide experience of the country who understand and sympathize with the people. The late President Nehru, in discussing this problem, pointed out that all existing knowledge is modern knowledge and there was no reason why Ayurvedic physicians should not have a basic training in modern scientific method. 'To him', as Professor Keswani has said, '*Dharma* (religion) was good so long as it did not come in conflict with a rational and scientific outlook. And fortunately for us, the hoary cultural heritage of India, imbued with philosophical ideas and religious beliefs that appeal to the fundamental unity of all in the basic Reality which is spiritual, and a comprehensiveness of outlook which knows no narrow distinctions, has never in its passage through the centuries, warranted war between theology and science.'

Laws are slow to change and it is practice rather than precept which has its impact on patients. We have to consider not only the restrictions which society imposes on the activities of the doctor, but also the changes in moral and ethical views which medicine induces in society.

In this connection it may be salutary to consider the views presented in a recent lecture by Lord Ritchie Calder. Discussing what has been called the 'population explosion' he calculated that, if present trends are allowed to continue unchecked, the earth's habitable areas would be so crowded by the middle of the next century that people would be forced to live in vast conurbations of 1,000 million inhabitants. This dreadful fate, which children born today might well live to endure, carried with it all the potentialities for famine, violence and insanity, and ultimate catastrophe. It was not, said Calder, a wild urge for procreation which had created this terrible dilemma, but the achievements of scientific medicine. Infant mortality had been drastically reduced, while life expectancy had been greatly increased. The great killing diseases which once took their regular toll of human life are now firmly under control, and we have been taught to take a pride in the triumphs of the medical scientists. They, like other scientists, are inclined to do whatever they find it possible to do, whether it be transplanting a young heart into an old body or devising ingenious instruments that will enable the babies terribly deformed by the action of modern drugs to survive into the age of what might come to be called human 'battery living'. Admiration for the technical expertise may temporarily blind us to the moral aspects of such activities. True, there has been a good deal of fuss about heart transplants, but chiefly because of the erroneous traditional view of the heart as the seat of the passions. The fundamental questions are rarely asked – at least in public – but if we are to avoid the ghastly prospect outlined for us by Ritchie Calder they must become the subject of profound and prolonged study and investigation. How much of our human resources – in wealth and other material goods and services, in intellectual and scientific manpower *ought* to be devoted – or even, can we *afford* to devote to ensuring the survival of congenital defectives or to prolonging the lives of old people which, without extraordinary measures, would already have come to a natural and peaceful end? These questions are loaded with moral and social implications. How could they be otherwise in a society whose current ethic is based on the Christian view of the sanctity of human life?

As a contribution to the discussion of these vital problems, the possible solutions to which will certainly affect all of us, it may be useful to look at other solutions which have been acceptable to societies at different periods of history and in different cultures.

As my historical case models, I propose to take abortion and the treatment of old people – circumstances associated with the beginning and the end of life – and in discussing these I shall of course have to allude to associated topics which affect the relationship between the doctor and society.

We shall start with the Greeks, for the earlier cultures took little note of this problem, except to lay down penalties for those who by deliberate or accidental violence were responsible for an abortion. Such penalties, as in the Hammurabi code of the Babylonians, were exacted to protect the rights of parents to their offspring who were regarded as gifts from the gods. In societies which needed children to maintain and increase a population, there was no particular shame attached to illegitimate birth and consequently no reason to seek desperate measures to end a pregnancy. The Mosaic code makes no mention of criminal abortion in our sense of the term.

When we consider the situation in Greece, we find that it begins with a paradox. The Hippocratic Oath, generally considered as a product of the fourth century B.C., although some scholars attribute it to Roman times and parts of it may be a thousand years later, seems to contain an unequivocal prohibition when the physician swears: 'I will not give to a woman an abortive remedy.'

Yet it is generally accepted that abortion was widely practised in Greece and Rome. Plato would even have had it made compulsory whenever the population of a state threatened to exceed the ideal number, or at any time if the potential mother was over 40. For eugenic reasons, this age ban on parenthood was extended to males over the age of 55 or so.

Aristotle made similar recommendations for limiting the population and even proposed a law forbidding any kind of care for infants with congenital defects. In Sparta, as you know, unwanted children were abandoned to the elements.

How can these facts be reconciled with the statement in the Hippocratic Oath? Twenty years ago, when Ludwig Edelstein published his erudite analysis of the Oath, he took this discrepancy between precept and practice as one of a number of quite strong arguments tending to prove that the Oath was of Pythagorean origin, for the followers of Pythagoras were the only Greek sect to disapprove of abortion. There is also the strange anomaly that in one of the Hippocratic books, which is acknowledged to be genuine, Hippocrates himself gives a case-history where a dancer who found herself pregnant and did not wish to give up her career sought his aid. He got her to jump up and down violently with her heels touching her buttocks each time, and after seven of these leaps the desired result was achieved. This fits in with what we know of the Greek attitude to abortion, but it is at variance with the Hippocratic Oath. It has been suggested that the Oath did not begin to be sworn by physicians until the first century of our era, when a strong movement developed towards strengthening the ethical principles of medical practice, a movement associated with the name of Scribonius

Largus and the Stoics. These points would be of academic interest only were it not for the fact that the Hippocratic Oath is still popularly supposed to be the ethical code of medical practice, although most of the medical professions of the world regard it as little more than a historical curiosity. How misplaced may be the popular confidence in the traditional merit of the Oath as a code of genuine ethics, rather than one of etiquette and protocol, is brought home to us whenever we try to elucidate its rather murky origins. Greek scholars have declared themselves unconvinced by Edelstein's arguments for a Pythagorean origin. If it is indeed Hippocratic, then force is added to the interpretation suggested by other commentators that this declaration is not in fact a ban on abortion, but an admission of a restrictive practice to avoid demarcation disputes. In Greek society obstetrics and gynaecology were generally dealt with by midwives, some of whom were expert and highly trained physicians and surgeons who occasionally wrote of the secrets of their craft. Literary evidence certainly bears out the view that by comparison with their knowledge, in these matters, that of the male physicians, even the greatest, was of small value. These women seem to have been skilled abortionists who were also able to advise their clients on effectual means of contraception. Against this background then, it has been suggested that the Oath merely records the male physicians' agreement not to meddle with such things but to leave it to the trained midwives.

One important matter came to be decided at this time in a way which was to affect the status of abortion for nearly two thousand years. In one of the Hippocratic writings it is stated that the shape of the child to be can be traced in the foetus at a very early stage, as early in fact as the seventh day. In another we are told that the foetus is inanimate until the 40th day, while contemporary and later writers fix this decisive event at the 60th or even as late as the 80th day. The comparative ignorance of the facts of foetal development is reflected in a traditional belief that it took 40 days for a male and 80 days for a female foetus to become animate. Both Plato and Aristotle recommend that abortion could safely be induced before this point was reached, and there are numerous references in the Hippocratic writings to abortion being advised when the foetus was 'silent' (i.e. immobile).

The existence of the mammalian ovum was not scientifically demonstrated until the nineteenth century, followed a decade or so later by the first observation (under a microscope) of its penetration by a spermatozoon. Hitherto the female role in conception was generally regarded as being limited to providing the nidus for the seed to develop, a belief that accorded well with early patriarchal societies. When we consider early laws about abortion we are not surprised to find then that they were designed to protect the father's rights in what was regarded as his property, to destroy or preserve as he wished. The mother, or any other person, had no right to make this decision for him, except perhaps the doctor if the mother's life was in danger should the pregnancy be allowed to go to full term. This was the position in Rome, as exemplified by a case quoted by Cicero, where an expectant mother had accepted money from her husband's heirs to produce an abortion. It was not the abortion *per se* which was criminal, but the conspiracy to deprive the husband of a natural heir.

There is ample evidence that abortion was commonplace in Imperial Rome, and allusions to it by Plautus, Ovid and other writers leaves us in no doubt that it was often resorted to for frivolous reasons. The rise of Christianity brought with it a religious viewpoint on abortion, or rather two viewpoints, for the old distinction between the formed and unformed foetus and the distinctive periods of forty and eighty days were still of great influence. They were accepted, for instance by Tertullian, who maintained, however, that 'to destroy the fruit of the mother in the womb, even when it is still unformed, is an "anticipated homicide"; for what difference is there between preventing the birth of a soul and destroying the body which that soul will animate? The man is within what one day will become a man, just as the fruit is in the seed.

Despite Tertullian, however, the laws laid down by a succession of Church councils, like St Augustine and Theodore, continued to make a practical distinction between the formed and the unformed foetus, for how could it be homicide to destroy an object without a soul? This distinction was reflected in the punishments, which ranged from fines or temporary excommunication for the abortion of an 'unformed' foetus to death for the homicide of a 'formed' foetus. Most commentators of these laws seem to have overlooked the medical conditions of the time which would have made it unlikely that abortion could be successfully induced halfway through a pregnancy without permanent harm to, or even the death of, the mother. May it have been in the minds of those who framed these laws that the death penalty would act as a deterrent to those who could so easily endanger a mother's life?

It is interesting to see that the same distinction between 'formed' and 'unformed' foetus is retained in the law of Charles V published in 1553.

This seems to have been the general situation with regard to abortion – a comparatively liberal and enlightened one, for abortion was not looked upon as a capital offence as long as it was restricted to the period while it was still comparatively harmless to the mother. This state of affairs was upset at the beginning of the seventeenth century, not by any sudden change of public opinion – although in a problem so closely linked with religion we cannot discount the influence of Reformation and Counter-reformation – but by the writings of one individual. This was a medical man named Thomas Fienus, who was born in Antwerp in 1567 and studied at the universities of Leyden and Bologna. He was called to occupy the first chair of medicine at Louvain and in 1620 he published at Antwerp a volume of 283 pages with the title: *On the formation of the foetus*, a book in which it is demonstrated that the rational soul is infused into it on the third day.

It sparked off a controversy, for it was seized upon by theologians and was attacked by other doctors, particularly by Louis du Gardin, professor of medicine at Douai, who published a penetrating criticism of Fienus's arguments. Fienus replied in another volume, was again attacked in print, this time by the physician to Philip IV, and again replied. So numerous and so complicated were his arguments that in 1629 he published a Synopsis of his three books on the subject. By this time, the theologians felt themselves in an impregnable position and employed the arguments advanced by Fienus to bring about a change in the laws. After a long run of something like two thousand years, the distinction between the inanimate and the animate foetus was abandoned, but not on grounds that we would today accept as scientific.

The laws of all modern European countries in the succeeding centuries were uncompromising about the criminal nature of voluntary abortion, yet the nature of the offence, and the lack of scientific knowledge to provide objective evidence of guilt, led to a widespread contempt of the law. It is generally acknowledged by jurists that a law which cannot be enforced is a bad law. The laws of a country are supposed to embody the views of its people on what is right and what is wrong. Yet, to take modern Britain alone, over the last century the estimated proportion of abortions to all pregnancies ranges from ten to twenty per cent. All authorities in this matter warn that it is impossible to produce reliable statistics, but these estimations are based on medical surveys made at various periods and are offered with the rider that they *must* be on the conservative side.

Until the recent Act, our own law was embodied in Sections 58 and 59 of the Offences against the Person Act, 1861, which was fairly typical of all European law until recent times. It imposes penalties up to penal servitude for life on a mother 'who uses poison or any other noxious thing, or shall unlawfully use any instrument or any other means whatsoever, with like intent, to procure a miscarriage ...' and the same penalties for any other found guilty of this same felony. The law was vague about therapeutic abortion, that is, when it was procured in order to save the life or health of the mother, and for over a century the only protection for the doctors who courageously intervened in this way was the one word 'unlawfully' in the Act – implying that there was some kind of undefined lawful abortion – and occasional assurances from legal luminaries that *of course* doctors would not be prosecuted for thus carrying out their medical duties. In fact, as we know, they occasionally were, and there have been one or two *causes célèbres* deliberately provoked as test cases.

There was another factor which disturbed the medical profession almost as much as the legal risk which they always incurred when considering medical interference with any pregnancy, and that was the activities of the back-street abortionists. These unqualified, inexpert and often unhygienic practitioners were the cause of a great number of maternal deaths. Moreover, recourse to their services tended to promote the popular use of untrained and inefficient doctors, a matter that was of great importance during the decades when the General Medical Council was attempting to repress unethical medical practice. What they were up against in this respect may be gauged from a cursory inspection of any selection of popular nineteenth-century newspapers and magazines, where numerous advertisements for thinly disguised abortifacients reflect the extent of the problem. We need not doubt the sincerity of the doctors' concern for this. The growth of scientific pharmacology in the nineteenth century had made it quite clear that there was in fact no safe abortifacient and that drugs employed for this purpose could only achieve their aim by doing harm, if only temporary harm.

The correspondence in *The Times* which preceded and accompanied the debates on the recent Act emphasizes the important role which the abortion problem has in the ethical framework of medical practice. The new Act was the product of almost a century's efforts to clarify the position. One of the many committees of various official bodies which investigated the problem was appointed by the B.M.A. on 25 July 1935, in response to a proposal passed by the representative body in 1933. It is worth looking at their published report rather closely. The reasons for the proposal are given as: '1. Medical practitioners were unwilling to perform therapeutic abortion owing to their sense of legal risk arising from the uncertain state of the law; and 2. That the medical profession should endeavour to guide public opinion, which was becoming more and more interested in this question.'

When the B.M.A. council reported back on this proposal in 1934 it stated that

On the question of guiding public opinion, the Council, after point-ing out that abortion was not solely a medical problem but one which was related also to the criminal law and to social, economic, ethical and religious standards and opinions, proceeded to express the fol-lowing views: 'While medical practitioners as citizens are entitled to hold individual opinions and cultivate activities on these several issues, the medical profession as such has no special right and no special competence to deal with them, and the Council therefore considers that any proposal that the profession ought to lead public opinion in such questions is one to be resisted. The medical profession in its corporate activities will best preserve its influence by keeping within the boundaries fixed by the particular expert technical knowledge of its members. If for legal, social, economic, ethical or religious reasons an inquiry on abortion is advisable, it is for those directly concerned to incur the responsibility and expense.

This view was accepted by the Annual Meeting of 1934, which set up the Committee to consider and report upon the medical aspects of abortion only.

Like so many Committee reports, this one offers fascinating reading between the lines. Paragraph 7 states:

The term 'abortion' is now generally applied to include all cases of expulsion of the foetus before the age of viability – that is, before 28 weeks or seven lunar months. The former practice by which 'abortion' was restricted to expulsion up to and including the 16th week, and 'miscarriage' to expulsion from the 16th to the 28th week, is now generally discarded in medical phraseology.

Surely we have here a reflection of the age-old argument about the 'unformed' and the 'formed' foetus. What is more, if we ask ourselves why at this point in time it became undesirable (or unnecessary?) to preserve the distinction, we may recall that the 1861 Act used only the term 'miscarriage'. Was it in this limitation and not only in the allusion to the 'unlawful procurement' that the doctor found his safety against prosecution? We may also recall that in 1929, just a few years earlier, there had been passed the Infant Life (Preservation) Act, the relevant clauses of which used neither the term 'abortion' nor 'miscarriage', but spoke simply of 'destroying the life of a child capable of being born alive'; adding that 'for the purposes of this Act, evidence that a woman had at any material time been pregnant for 28 weeks or more shall be *prima facie* proof that she was at the time pregnant of a child capable of being born alive.'

Here it was explicitly stated that 'no person shall be found guilty of an offence under this section unless it is proved that the act which caused the death of the child was not done in good faith for the purpose only of preserving the life of the mother.'

This seems to give clear permission for therapeutic abortion, but dissatisfaction with the 'vagueness of the law' is expressed in the Committee's report of 1936. Paragraph 17 admits that the law is in fact adaptable in practice, although not in theory, to changes in social thought. To this argument (it continues) it may be replied that it is unfair to place upon the doctor the responsibility of interpreting public opinion on such matters.

Whatever the medical profession, in its corporate capacity, may think about its ability to guide or influence public opinion, the fact remains that scientifically based medical practice, both curative and preventive, has so changed the social conditions that people will be forced to change their opinions, and governments be forced to change their laws, if either people or government is to survive.

The so-called permissive societies of Western Europe have in the last few years allowed unprecedented freedom of discussion in all the mass media on methods of oral contraception. The pill has brought about a situation where no enlightened society would tolerate any kind of laws forbidding its use; or if such laws were ever passed they would be impossible to enforce. At the same time, the great advances in biochemistry which have made it possible to devise the almost perfect contraceptive have also produced drugs which cure sterility. Their use carries the risk of promoting multiple births and the same issue of the newspaper or the same news bulletin which shows children starving in Africa, or which reports concern about the population explosion and demands energetic measures to cope with it in India, has excited accounts of the birth of quintuplets in Birmingham or Sydney, whilst the mother is treated to the same kind of publicity as is usually accorded to the winners of the big prizes in the football pools. If these organs of public opinion, these moulders of opinion, are so confused in their outlook, how can we expect the masses of the people to have any clear and consistent viewpoint on this matter?

It may be argued that, however many mouths there may be to feed in the world, man's ingenuity is such that he can always invent new ways of creating food, new resources to exploit, as the oceans are now beginning to be exploited. This may well be so, but there is still the problem of living space. When it comes to the crunch, it seems likely that the problem of abortion, which has been one of the central features of medical ethics for over two thousand years, will be removed entirely from any ethical context. I am not quoting science fiction, but quoting from a conversation among research scientists when I say that it is highly probable that the day will come, and sooner rather than later, when one of the chemical additives to the staple food of all peoples will be an oral contraceptive, and that those privileged couples whom the State allows to have children will be prescribed a special pill to counteract the effects of the contraceptive for a predetermined period. I must leave it to students of the contemporary political scene to give their own estimates of the length of time required for the United Nations, or any other international body, to come to any effective agreement on such a universal measure, and of the tremendous instinctive reaction that even the hint of such a proposal would arouse in many Western countries. We can all discuss quietly and objectively what is best for the Indians or the Chinese, but are less receptive to the same proposals for ourselves.

In these questions of demography history must provide the case records for our findings, and our own demographic historians have tended to argue that food supply was the over-riding factor in our own population changes, that medical advances and public health measures have played a very small part. Even if this were true for the nineteenth century, which seems unlikely, there are powerful arguments for the contrary today. Writing in the Lancet on 'Medical Ethics and Social Change in Developing Countries', Professor Titmuss reported what has become a classic study of the island of Mauritius. 'Until 1947', he writes, 'it could hardly be said that Mauritius had a population problem. Then the World Health Organization and teams of scientists from Britain intervened to control malaria. Since then the rate of growth has been phenomenal – well over 3 per cent per year, and one of the highest (if not the highest) in the world. It took Britain nearly fifty years to halve her infant-mortality rate. Mauritius has done it in less than five years. . . . Population control in the form of family limitation is essential for economic growth. In the time available it is the only non-violent answer to the threat of population disaster.'

A contribution made to a recent symposium by the Indian Ambassador to the United States offers further evidence from those who are close to the problem. He writes:

At one time a rising population did not present a serious problem in India. There were always epidemics, or local wars or a heavy infant mortality and a low expectancy of life to counterbalance the large number of births. I may also point out that people in those days looked upon a large number of children as an insurance – so few survived that a large family seemed to be essential. But all that has changed now. Advance in medical knowledge, steps taken to improve standards of hygiene have eliminated many diseases in India which took a heavy toll of lives. There are no epidemics now, and if one breaks out it can immediately be put down. Civilization no longer believes in small local wars – we have to wait for a nuclear holocaust. The result has been a sharp fall in the death rate. But the birth rate has remained the same. So in a sense we have been suffering from the civilizing effects of science and medical research. Civilization has shown us how to reduce our death rate but so far has failed to point the way to a controlled population. I think this is one of the most important issues of conscience in modern medicine. Medicine must advance on both the fronts. If it considers life is sacred and everything must be done to prolong it, it must also prevent human beings being born into an existence of poverty, destitution and frustration. The sanctity of life demands that the dignity of the individual must be upheld. What dignity will millions of children have who are being born into the world today?

In these last two sentences we have the real kernel of the problem. Society is faced with a dilemma which the conflicts between its own social mores and religious beliefs make it almost impossible to resolve *in time* and so puts the burden of choice on the doctor. Medicine is responsible for this dilemma, for it has destroyed the normal biological checks and balances; therefore medicine must find the way out. We also have the cue to another problem, the treatment of the aged. 'Life is sacred, and everything must be done to prolong it.'

We live in a country with a steadily increasing proportion of old people, so here again we have a situation in which we are all, whether we like it or not, intimately and perhaps more immediately involved. Starting again from the contemporary scene, we might ask ourselves if we are justified in placing upon the medical profession the very great ethical strains implicit in the hospitalization of the chronic sick, most of whom have already passed the average life-span. The scientific resources of modern medicine have made it possible to extend such lives, and because it is now *possible*, the doctor *must* do so, even if his own conscience and common sense prompt him otherwise. The pattern of family life in this country has changed in such a way in the present century that younger members are no longer prepared to accept the burden of caring for their own sick and old. Any practitioner in the National Health Service can cite numerous instances of the stubborn repudiation of this obligation, which therefore becomes the duty of the State welfare services. Once they are in hospital, it is the doctor's ethical duty to prolong their life as long as possible.

Such cases already comprise a very large proportion of the hospital population, placing a very great strain on the human and physical resources available to the Health Service. Now and again there is an outcry in the press when the service breaks down under this strain and falls below the level considered decent in a humane society. But the true nature of the problem is rarely exposed, that the richest country in the world could not afford to devote to its solution all the human and financial resources necessary to solve it now and to prevent its constant recurrence in the future. The choice is being made pragmatically now by what are in fact economic sanctions by the State, while the doctor is left to carry the ethical burden as best he may. Meantime, sensational publicity is given in the mass media to new scientific techniques and complicated and expensive apparatus designed to keep the human body alive long after the will, and even the independent capacity to live, has left it. Expensive research is undertaken into the problems of ageing and into means of prolonging life, yet if one talks very much to old people one meets very few who are not able to contemplate their own approaching dissolution with tranquillity and who do not feel, when at last in hospital and 'everything possible is being done' in their last few weeks or days, that these urgent attentions are an intrusion and an affront to their intelligence and their human dignity.

Let us go over briefly what has happened in other periods and other cultures in these circumstances.

Among primitive societies generally, the very old and the

dying were regarded with emotions ranging from the highest honour and veneration – for their influence with the gods whom they were about to meet could be of benefit to the tribe – to fear and degradation. Agricultural communities with a fixed food supply often abandoned their old people to starve, and in some tribes the old had the right to request death.

If we look at the situation in India, we find in the Upanishads that when a man became old (and this was placed as early as 40 years of age) he should leave his family and live as a hermit devoted to the study of the sacred books and renouncing all earthly pleasures.

There is one relevant passage which is worth quoting:

> He should not wish to die,
>   nor hope to live,
> but await the time appointed,
>   as a servant awaits his wages . . .
> Rejoicing in the things of the Spirit, calm,
>   caring for nothing, abstaining from sensual pleasure,
> himself his only helper,
>   he may live on in the world, in the hope of eternal bliss

This kind of mysticism was alien to the Greeks, who feared and detested old age because of the sickness it brought and the decay of physical and intellectual powers. The Athenian laws made it obligatory for sons to care for their aged and infirm parents and respect for the old was inculcated in youth. Plato declared that it is better to die than to live in sickness, while Aristotle asserted that nobody could consider the old happy, for they have to abstain from all or nearly all of the pleasures of life. Euripides, in a judgement endorsed by Plutarch on those who patiently endure long illness, wrote:

> I hate the men who would prolong their lives
> By food and drinks and charms of magic art,

> Perverting Nature's course to keep off death;
> They ought, when they no longer serve the land,
> To quit this life and clear the way for youth.

Resort was often had to suicide, especially in cases of blindness, and it was regarded as an honourable and virtuous end to life. The Hippocratic writings made frequent mention of the hopeless cases which the physician should not treat, and it was probably true then, as it certainly was in the later classical period, that a patient would have felt tricked if the doctor had not told him the truth about his condition. He had to make his will and settle his affairs with his family, and when the end came he wished to die calmly and nobly as befits a man. To the supposed founder of medical ethics, the question 'Should a doctor tell?' would have seemed an extraordinary question.

These remarks must be reserved of course for the Greek or Roman *citizen*; the fate of elderly and sick slaves depended entirely on the character of their master. Some were sold off cheaply as today old horses are disposed of; others were just abandoned, in Roman times in such numbers that the Emperor Claudius set aside an island in the Tiber as a refuge for them, where any that recovered could claim their freedom. This island has often been cited as the first general hospital.

Among the Roman writers we find already in Lucretius the view that ageing and death are an essential part of the natural order to prevent over-population, while Cicero thought of death as the 'goal of life', when the soul would be released from its bodily prison.

And here begins the long and familiar Christian belief that life on this earth is but the prelude to an immortal life hereafter. The good Christian never fears death. St Paul tells us, 'My desire is to depart and be with Christ, for that is far better', and 'The last enemy to be destroyed is death'. St Augustine believed that all human existence was striving towards eternal life, while Thomas Aquinas combines Aristotle's view of death as an essential stage in the natural order of things with the Christian view of death as punishment for the sin of Adam.

Throughout the Christian centuries, both doctors and priests have been concerned that those for whom they cared should have a 'good' death, and innumerable religious tracts and sermons survive from all periods testifying to the skill and compassion with which believers were helped to face what was for them an end and a beginning. Since birth and death were matters of concern to both doctor and priest, we find a certain dualism in the attitude of the doctor as he begins to glimpse the possibilities opened up by science. In this connection it is interesting to find that Descartes, in his great *Discourse*, confesses that his own medical studies had been embarked upon with the idea of finding ways of alleviating the disabilities of age and prolonging life.

All at present known in medicine [he wrote] is almost nothing in comparison with what remains to be discovered . . . We could free ourselves from an infinity of maladies of body as well as mind, and perhaps also even from the debility of age, if we had sufficiently ample knowledge of their causes, and of all the remedies provided for us by nature.

And in a letter to Constantine Huyghens he wrote:

It seems to be evident that if we guard ourselves from certain errors which we customarily commit in our way of life, we will be able without other inventions to achieve an old age much longer and happier than now.

Descartes was unsuccessful in his own efforts to prolong his life, for he died at the age of 54. In the *Discourse* he compared philosophy to a tree with three branches – mechanics, medicine, and ethics; and he believed that medicine was the foundation of ethics, the object of which, as he declares elsewhere in the book, is 'to teach men to submit to the world as it is'.

It is perhaps significant that here, at the very heart of one of the foundation stones of modern science and the scientific outlook there is buried a paradox. The movement to which Descartes gave its early impetus has brought more changes in the world, and in the life of man, than he could ever have imagined. The ethics, which he truly saw to be so closely associated with medicine, still has its mission of teaching man to submit to the world as it is, while all around is changing so rapidly that we lose sight of the purpose. We must at least see clearly, if not submit to, the world as it is before we can plan a future which has any kind of meaning.

5

Medicine and Philosophy

ONE of Aristotle's tenets was that 'The philosopher must begin with medicine, and the physician must end with philosophy'. This aphorism may mislead modern readers, for philosophy to Aristotle had a much wider connotation than it has today and included all the field of knowledge and inquiry now covered by the term 'science' and at one time by the term 'natural philosophy'. Morals and metaphysics were a part of traditional philosophy, and Aristotle wrote of these too, as well as of logic and poetry. As the greatest biologist of antiquity, Aristotle came to hold a central place in the development of medical and scientific thought, holding that the way to discovery lay in observation and experience. In contrast, his own teacher Plato held that truth could only be known by divine revelation after contemplation of the object, a belief that was endorsed by Augustine and held sway until St Thomas Aquinas based his *Summa*, or account of all that was known at his time, on Aristotle's philosophy. As far as medical knowledge was concerned, this change fitted in well with the views of the greatest authority in this field, Galen, the second-century Greek physician who became physician to the emperor Marcus Aurelius. He succeeded in bringing together into a single system all that was worth while in the medical writings of the preceding five centuries and in his writings Aristotelianism is all-pervasive.

Aristotle and Galen provided the structure for the development of Islamic science and medicine from the eighth to the twelfth centuries with Averroes and Avicenna as their respective exponents, and their writings had the greatest influence on the West when they were brought into Europe in Latin versions. Padua in particular became a great stronghold of Aristotelianism and it was there that William Harvey, while a medical student, was first put upon the path which led him to discover the circulation of the blood. Many commentators have described the little book in which he announced his discovery in 1628 as the first demonstration of modern scientific method and consequently the 'corner-stone' of modern science, but as Walter Pagel has clearly shown, Harvey's approach to the problem was clearly Aristotelian. That the apparent conflict between these two views may be reconciled is a possibility when we find the present Director of the National Institute of Medical Research, Sir Peter Medawar, suggesting that the pattern of discovery in scientific research is still essentially Aristotelian. It is certainly true that the results of Aristotle's own investigations in natural science, for example, on the parts of animals, have far more in common with modern scientific work on the same topics than have Plato's almost mystical speculations on anatomy and physiology in his *Timaeus*.

However, few scientists today would acknowledge that they hold to any philosophy in any formal sense of the term. Their search for the accumulation and verification of objective facts has a 'dehumanizing' effect which makes many non-scientists uneasy to the point of hostility. When science is applied to the particular needs of medicine, where the human being, the patient, is the centre of interest, it may often be found wanting. Because of the great transformation which the application of the basic sciences has brought about in modern medicine it is fashionable to talk of 'scientific medicine', where any philosophy is repudiated as mere speculation. Yet many practising physicians feel the need for it, realizing that any number of scientific facts established by experiments and supported by statistics, however true they may be of man in the abstract, may not be true of Mr X or Mrs Y. That this same need is felt even in framing the broader policies of health care is indicated by a recent letter in the *Lancet* in which the correspondent deplores 'the lack of definition of a basic philosophy of health which would make it possible to rationalize the allocation of limited means to unlimited ends. Medicine is an instrument of social policy but mere juggling with facts will not provide a solution. What we do not have is a coherent theory of the relationship between the multitude of facts and the achievement of health, which is the object of the service'.

The definition of a 'basic philosophy of health' in this context involves far more than any abstraction derived from medical and scientific thought and practice, for it brings in also the social responsibility for all this activity and the political and economic theories which affect it. Although in practice medical care almost everywhere is based on the assumption that health is the absence of disease, most doctors would repudiate any such negative definition. This repudiation would be the reaction of intelligent and educated men and women rather than a response conditioned by any part of their professional training, which is almost entirely orientated towards the discovery and treatment of defect and disorder rather than towards positive health, however this may be defined.

Many patients with experience of hospital investigations resulting in a verdict of 'no pathology' would also be reluctant to accept such a definition. A patient with 'no pathology' may still feel ill and in some cases a psychiatrist may eventually reveal that the *malaise* has its source in personal frustrations, domestic tensions or work in a job which gives little or no satisfaction. None of these can be treated by a doctor in a busy out-patient clinic, although they undoubtedly prevent the patient from enjoying positive good health. Some doc-

tors, and many patients, look back to some past age when, we
are told, the doctor was family friend and counsellor as well
as physician who could help his patients to achieve the 'good
life'. If such a relationship ever existed in more than a few
individual instances it was enjoyed by only a minute proportion of the population of any country, and it is one which
could not be applied in any system of mass medical care
current today.

Before we can begin to define any 'basic philosophy of
health', we may well wonder whether the doctor is being
asked to carry the burden of failure in the 'body politic' rather
than to treat the disorder of the affected individual. It is often
said that with the decline of popular belief in any organized
religion, the doctor has taken the place of the priest. If this is
so, then it is a role which the doctor has not sought and for
which he is not trained. In the days before medicine was as
scientific as it is today, the doctor enjoyed a certain 'mystique'
upon which he depended for much of the good which it was
within his power to do his patients. Like the medicine man in
a primitive tribe, he too employed ritual gestures and ritual
phrases which reassured and comforted. In these egalitarian
days he has been robbed of most of his mystique by those who
are sceptical of anything which cannot be weighed and
measured. He is reminded that medicine is 'just a job', a technology employing a variety of technical skills. It is therefore
illogical to express disappointment that the doctor can no
longer play the part of the medicine man, ministering to the
mind as well as the body. It is also illogical to suggest that such
a technology should have any concern with philosophy, any
more than has engineering or accountancy.

Nevertheless, the situation in which we now find ourselves
is a transient one which has itself been brought about by
philosophies of one kind or another acting over very long
periods on medicine itself and on the society in which medi-

cine is practised. For more than 2,000 years the prevailing concept of disease was that based on the ancient Greek notions of the elements, earth, air, fire and water, from which all things are formed, mediated by a fifth, all pervasive substance called ether. Corresponding to the four elements were the four qualities, dry, cold, hot and moist. Following the same pattern, there were four humours in the body, blood, phlegm, yellow bile and black bile. Blood was hot and moist; phlegm was cold and moist; yellow bile was hot and dry; black bile was cold and dry. Perfect health depended upon the balance of these humours and disease was caused when this natural balance was temporarily disturbed. A whole system of pathology was built up on this basis; different organs and different diseases were classified according to these categories, and even drugs came to be arranged on the same principles, so that a remedy that was hot and dry was prescribed for a disease which was cold and moist.

The theoretical nature of such a system fitted perfectly into an age which delighted in logical, theological and philosophical systems, and so familiar was it as a way of thought that nobody ever dreamed of questioning its validity. Some historians see in it a foreshadowing of our modern ideas of metabolic disorders and of the importance of biochemistry in physiology and pathology. Whether it is or not, the humoral doctrine has certainly left its mark on our civilization. We still speak of good humour and bad humour, and of a man's temperament or complexion. Of these also there were four, according to the innate preponderance or dominance of one or other of the humours; the sanguine (blood), hot and moist; the choleric (yellow bile), hot and dry; the phlegmatic (phlegm), cold and moist; and the melancholy (black bile), cold and dry. Even classes, professions and occupations were arranged in a hierarchy according to these same qualities, and here the doctor is found to be properly under the influence of the planet Mars, his dominant humour yellow bile (hot and dry), and his temperament choleric.

Here then was a medical philosophy which suited both doctors and patients. It fitted in with the divine order of things, with balance and imbalance, harmony and discord, health and disease, as basic and linked concepts. It provided a body of scientific knowledge for the profession of medicine which required learning and skill in its application. The usual treatments – the removal of the 'peccant' humours by purgation and blood-letting – were appreciated and easily understood by the patients, even when they were taken to heroic extremes, and despite them many patients recovered, even from serious illnesses. If they did not, then it was the divine will. All were satisfied that 'everything possible had been done'.

This system was part of that natural philosophy without which, said Bacon, the science of medicine 'is not much better than an empirical practice'. In Bacon's time an 'empiric' (i.e. an empirical practitioner) was synonymous with a charlatan whose treatments were not designed or applied 'according to art', that is, the basic philosophy (or science) on which the 'art' of medicine was based. Despite his apparent condemnation of empiricism, Bacon removed medicine from the sphere of natural philosophy and gave it a special category of its own as knowledge concerned with man's body only, as distinct from mind. He considered that more would be learned about the body and its working by careful study without any preconceived ideas or *a priori* hypotheses and that when enough facts about it had been accumulated then some more general explanation would be possible. The potentialities of such an approach to research were already obvious in the new and flourishing science of anatomy which received its impetus from the work of Vesalius in the sixteenth century. Objective observation of structure had replaced tradition and written authority as a path to knowledge, and the same kind of observation had enabled Fabricius to demonstrate the valves in the veins, which first gave William Harvey his idea of the circulation of the blood, which he proved by 'ocular demonstration'.

Reinforcing the Baconian accumulation of factual observations came the new methodology that sprang from the Galilean revolution in physics. Weighing and measuring gave precision to sense impressions and one of Galileo's pupils, Sanctorius, devised a weighing machine for measuring the loss of body weight by invisible perspiration as well as a clinical thermometer, and a pendulum for measuring the pulse rate. Harvey also measured the amount of blood which the heart could hold as well as its output in each contraction and used his results in the triumphant conclusion of his demonstration.

In 1628, when Harvey's book was published, just two years after Bacon's death, the young Descartes was already planning his career in philosophy which was to have a profound influence on medical thought. Primarily a mathematician, Descartes sought a mechanical explanation of every phenomenon and made mathematics the basis of his method. According to him, the human body is a complicated machine designed by God and infused by a 'rational soul'. He located the centre of activity of this soul as the pineal gland but it was not susceptible to the same kind of investigation as the body. If we ignore the misguided attempt to locate the seat of the soul, Descartes' idea of the 'rational soul' permeating and directing the body is not so far from Aristotle's final belief that soul and body are a natural and indivisible whole, the soul being the source of the body. It is worth recalling this fact to remind us that no philosophy or body of ideas is ever completely ousted by another, but strands of the one persist and eventually influence the other.

Although Descartes' 'rational soul' was brought in as the mainspring, as it were, of the divine clockwork, it was not a spring that could be weighed or measured, and the assumption of its existence did not interfere with the piecemeal investigation of the parts which were so cunningly brought together in the whole body. Moreover, since he postulated that the lower animals had no soul and were therefore merely some kind of physical automata, the working of organs and their interrelated effects could be studied by experiments on living animals. Although this was no novelty, and although there are no precise records for purposes of comparison, we have the impression that these greatly increased in number in the later decades of the seventeenth century and were often used to good effect, as in de Graaf's study of the pancreas and its secretions.

In England the 'new philosophy' was regarded more sceptically, and although the Royal Society in its early decades energetically explored every new idea and scientific report in pursuing its aim to develop new sciences, it was not until Newton's *Principia* appeared in 1687 that a new school of 'mathematical and mechanical physicians' began to develop there. One of the most important and earliest results of the Cartesian approach was Borelli's demonstration of muscular action (Rome, 1680), but Stephen Hales's first attempt to measure blood pressure (1733) was based entirely on Newtonian principles.

There were 'iatrochemists' as well as 'iatromechanists', and these were strongly influenced by Paracelsus and Van Helmont, who believed that chemistry could provide the answer to most medical questions. It was Van Helmont who first identified acid digestion in the stomach and who coined the term 'gas'. Belonging to neither school was the English clinician Thomas Sydenham who, in the long run, was to have a greater impression on English medicine than either.

Like Descartes, he was not a great reader and he shared with the great French philosopher a scant respect for authority. He studied the problems of disease as a naturalist studies plants or animals, accumulating facts from observation in the Baconian manner until he was able to differentiate certain patterns or symptoms which were always associated with certain diseases. In this way, he was able to identify clearly scarlet fever, rheumatic fever, and gout, and to chart their natural course through onset, crisis and resolution. Sydenham also, like Hippocrates, with whom he was often compared, studied epidemics and what he called 'epidemic constitutions', keeping careful records in an attempt to correlate the rise and fall of epidemics with weather and seasons.

Of even greater influence was the work of Robert Boyle, who was at the centre of the group which formed the Royal Society. Although primarily a chemist, his investigations ranged over the whole field of science and even into medicine and physiology. Resisting the mechanical philosophy of Descartes, he was greatly impressed by the revival of Greek atomism led by another French philosopher Pierre Gassendi who taught that atomic or 'corpuscular' motion provided a sufficient explanation of all physical phenomena. This theory is much in evidence in Boyle's inquiries into the action of specific medicines (1685). Because the Galenic system could offer no rational explanation of this, many physicians refuted the possibility of any specific drug, and this at a time when cinchona bark (from which quinine was later extracted) was already being shown to be effective against malaria. In his attempt to resolve these difficulties Boyle had recourse to atomism, declaring that 'the human body is an engine' and that it contains 'many strainers (i.e. organs)' and 'divers ferments'. Carried around by the blood, the specific is changed and 'the medicine (crumbled as it were in minute corpuscles) arrives at the part or humour to be wrought upon' and so is able to 'restore the tone or texture of the strainers, or alter the blood, or resolve and carry away such tenacious matter, as stuffed or choaked up the slender passages of the strainer, or at least straitened its pores, or vitiated their figure.'

In this brief passage we can discern several competing philosophical theories together with the old Galenism and the new physiology of Harvey, reminding us that there is never any clear-cut point of departure in the history of ideas but rather a gradual merging of new ideas into old and a gradual separating out and abandonment of old standpoints as new facts are accumulated which require an explanation. The facts alone, without the explanation, are never entirely satisfactory, and sometimes the explanation may be long deferred, as in Jenner's empirical demonstration of the prophylactic value of vaccination against smallpox, for it was more than a century before the new science of immunology provided a scientific explanation.

Here then, already by the end of the seventeenth century and influenced by the flood of new ideas which characterized this period of great scientific change, we see trends which have become prominent more than two centuries later. Experimental physiology, pharmacology, biochemistry, biophysics on the one side, all probing more and more minutely into the organs and tissues of the body and their functions, and on the other, as a counterbalance, an attempt by the physician to retain a comprehensive and integrating view of the whole.

Developments in medicine in those intervening centuries show, when we regard them with hindsight, that although physicians eagerly embraced philosophical theories, as if they needed intellectual reassurance that what they were doing was right, the methods most productive of genuinely new and useful knowledge were those of Bacon rather than Descartes. John Locke, in his *Essay concerning Human Understanding*, emphasized the limitations of philosophical inquiry and gave added force to an empirical approach which has often been considered as characteristically English in its distrust of speculation and plausible explanations. His approach to medical problems is typified by the work of his friend, Thomas Sydenham, and yet Sydenham became one of the guiding stars of the great Dutch clinician Hermann Boerhaave, who dominated medical thought for the greater part of the eighteenth century. Unfortunately, Boerhaave's authority rested upon a system of medicine based on an eclectic philosophy which owed much to all the ideas that emerged in the seventeenth century. It was unfortunate because it accepted and welded them all together with a bold assurance which contrasted greatly with the humility and caution of a man like Locke.

To practising physicians, Boerhaave seemed to know the answer to most of their questions. He was very learned, and philosophy was his first study before he went on to medicine. At Leyden he held three chairs, in botany, chemistry and medicine, and he introduced the teaching of students at the bedside in the hospital there, so stressing the importance of clinical observation in the manner of Sydenham. His influence spread to Edinburgh and Vienna, both of which became leading centres of medical ideas. Among much that was good in his teaching there was much that went far beyond his own precepts of observation and experience into the realm of speculation where surmise was presented as fact.

One celebrated but equally erroneous theory which replaced Boerhaave's teaching was that formulated by John Brown, an Edinburgh-trained physician who produced an idea that we may now regard as a caricature of all philosophically based theories of medicine. Drawing on physiological views current at the time, especially Stahl's vitalism and Haller's ideas of the 'irritability' of tissues, Brown put forward the idea that the body possessed a general 'excitability' and that all diseases were caused by a deficiency or excess of this principle. They were therefore classified as 'asthenic' or 'sthenic', the former being treated by stimulants and a rich diet, the latter by sedatives and a low diet. He published an account of his system in Latin in 1780 and soon thousands of physicians in Europe were practising according to 'the Brunonian system', his book being translated into Italian, French, German and Spanish.

Of more lasting significance was the fact that at this time the famous French *Encyclopédie* in which Diderot and his associates surveyed the whole of human knowledge presented Medicine as a part of the natural sciences, so vindicating Sydenham, whose influence was still alive in France among the pre-revolutionary philosophers. The revolution itself brought about a breakdown in the old type of family medicine and a great change in the training of doctors, for the old university medical faculties were abolished and training centred in the hospitals. In these conditions, where patients were assembled in close proximity for treatment, there was ample evidence supporting Sydenham's views of symptom patterns and disease entities. In consequence, it became easier for the doctor to study objectively the natural history of particular diseases and to give precision to the physical signs by which its presence could be diagnosed.

Combined with the new type of scientific pathology which replaced the old humoral pathology when the Italian Morgagni demonstrated the location of disease in particular organs by correlating case records with post mortem reports, the French clinicians were able to bring scientific method to the bedside. In doing so, the disease rather than the patient became the subject of treatment. In short, the patient became 'a case'. Since it was not possible to make a visual examination of the liver, or the heart, or the lungs, in the living subject, efforts were made to visualize the state of these organs by new diagnostic aids. The process began with percussion and Laennec's stethoscope, to be followed by many other kinds of 'scopes' to enable the clinician to see the interior of organs and body cavities, reinforced by the microscopical study of tissues, blood and other body fluids, by chemical tests, and eventually by radiology and radioactive isotopes used as tracers. The success of this line of inquiry has been demonstrated over and over again and many doctors today would agree with the statement made a century ago by Claude Bernard that 'philosophy does not teach anything, and it is unable to teach anything by itself since philosophy makes neither experiments nor observations'.

This may well be true if we equate philosophy with metaphysics and theology, but one of the fashionable philosophies of Bernard's day was the positivist philosophy of Auguste Comte, which he presented as the historical successor of theology and metaphysics. For his investigation of man in society, Comte advocated the use of that scientific method which was proving so successful in the laboratory to elucidate problems in chemistry and physiology, observing and analysing phenomena and classifying them with related phenomena. His 'social physics' expounded 'laws of progress' which seemed self-evident to men engaged in adding considerably to the world's material goods by new industries and manufactures. The utilitarian philosophers who drew their inspiration from Jeremy Bentham (who was a great practical reformer rather than a philosopher) also used the methods of science for investigating and accumulating information about social phenomena, but with much greater effect. To their group belonged Edwin Chadwick and Thomas Southwood Smith, who were respectively Bentham's secretary and medical adviser, and between them they began that comprehensive inspection of social evils which undermined the health of the people and led the campaigns of reform which resulted in public health legislation. In his original 'Constitutional Code', Bentham had postulated the necessity for a Minister of Health and listed in detail all the national and local health institutions and agencies required to guard the people's health. It took a century to realize his programme fully, and its realization is a memorial to his principle of 'the greatest happiness for the greatest number'.

While the organization of social medicine based on these ideas was being systematically developed in Britain and some other highly industrialized countries, another philosophy, inspired by the work of Karl Marx, was to take over from the utilitarians as a source of reforming energy. Reversing the order of Hegel's triad of thought, nature and matter, the followers of Marx have developed a creed called 'dialectical materialism' in which all human needs and interests are subjugated to materialist ends. Undistinguished by subtlety of thought or originality, for it was merely a by-product of Marx's economic and social analysis, it made 'economic man' the central feature and it would have had little effect on man's intellectual history if it had not become the official doctrine of the Soviet Union and of the political adherents of communism throughout the world.

Its effect on medicine in the Soviet Union is seen largely in the sphere of social medicine, and here disinterested observers find a well organized and maintained system of medical care, with particular attention being paid to maternity and child welfare clinics, local health centres and occupational health. In contrast to the United States, a large proportion of the medical personnel are women and in the field of routine medical care (as opposed to medical and scientific research, where rewards are often higher than in the West) remuneration is little higher than that of the skilled artisan.

It has also resulted in the development of a special 'Marxist science', the manipulation of which for political ends has occasionally led to controversy with Western scientists, as in the notorious Lysenko case, where older Lamarckian theories of inheritance of acquired characteristics (as interpreted by Lysenko) were officially preferred to the genetic principles elucidated by Mendel and his followers. The work of Pavlov on conditioned reflexes, carried out in Tsarist Russia and in no way influenced by Marxist ideas, also fitted in well with official doctrine in the Soviet Union as well as with the scientific determinism current elsewhere. It has been adopted as the basis of a growing 'behaviourist school' of psychology which holds that trained reflexes explain all facets of human behaviour and that mind and the unconscious may for all practical purposes be ignored, a doctrine which is of obvious significance in psychiatry. Opposed to Freudian analysis with its metaphysical and almost mystical aspects, it is clearly better suited to mass application and seems a logical consequence of the growth of knowledge in neurology and psychosomatic medicine.

Appreciation of the fact that the mind acts upon the body and can produce physical disorders was always an important part of medical knowledge and is as old as Galen. This seems to have been forgotten in the nineteenth century and was 're-discovered' after the work of Pavlov and Freud had had its effect, although as early as 1870 a British pioneer in psychiatry, Henry Maudsley, published a book on the relationship between mind and body in the causation of mental illness and repudiated the positivist philosophy of Comte as an exploitation of science for unworthy ends. The isolation of 'lunatics' in 'asylums' in the nineteenth century tended to keep mental illness out of the mainstream of medical advance. The ancient methods of forcible restraint in the treatment of the insane were generally abandoned, but it was taken for granted that little could be done to cure them until neurology and neurosurgery indicated a more hopeful direction. The National

Hospital for Nervous Diseases in London began as a small hospital for the paralysed and the epileptic in 1859, a place of refuge for patients not accepted in other hospitals. It grew into a world centre which led to the development of a new medical science in the light of which many mental disorders have been shown to originate in physical conditions and to respond to physical treatment. The demonstration that the surgeon's knife or the use of certain drugs could restore mental balance has provided additional support for behaviourists and others who assert that if you look after the body the mind will look after itself.

The operation of pre-frontal lobotomy on the brain, introduced in the 1930s but no longer favoured, turns a potentially dangerous mentally disturbed patient into an acquiescent and passive observer of the human scene and is only one of many physical methods now available for changing human personality. From ancient times, and even among so-called 'primitive' tribes, it has been known that certain drugs can bring about changes in personality. In the last 25 years a great range of new drugs has been made accessible to the physician for this purpose following the trial use of an extract from a plant (*rauwolfia*) which has been used in indigenous Indian medicine for over a thousand years to treat the mentally ill. Any drug is a two-edged weapon and some which have been most effective in emptying the old asylums of their long-stay patients have also been abused to create a drug problem among the youth of many countries who seek to escape from a society where materialist values are dominant. There seems little doubt that drugs have also been used to reinforce suggestion in the so-called 'brain-washing' for political purposes.

Meanwhile, many other sciences have contributed to the belief that all life can be explained in terms of 'matter in motion'. In the time of Descartes man was distinguished from the lower animals by the possession of a 'rational soul', and the evolutionist theories of Darwin and his followers were bitterly attacked by the theologians for their implication that man was distinguished from other animals only by a larger brain, by the erect posture and by the ability to use his hands. They also seemed to replace the divine will by random chance and blind necessity, aspects which were unlikely to recommend them to practising physicians, although they undoubtedly gave an impetus to medical and biological research based on the concept of man as part of nature and susceptible to all the methods of inquiry open to the natural scientist. In this research animals were employed and vivisection was not uncommon, much to the distress of many people in England who began to endow animals with 'souls' just as man was, scientifically, losing his own.

A further argument for the materialist was provided by the revelation of 'germs' as the final causes of many diseases. Epidemics that were once thought to be a punishment from God were seen to be the result of human failure and ignorance. And when the ordinary microscope had ranged through the whole gamut of microscopic life there came the electron microscope to carry on the same task with viruses, some of which have been found to be almost indistinguishable from chemical structures. Mendel's work on the laws of inheritance had been published just before the dawn of the science of bacteriology, but remained unknown to the scientific world until the turn of the century. From it have grown the investigations of genes and chromosomes and the dawn of a new science called 'genetic engineering', recalling Boyle's definition of the body of man as a 'hydraulico-pneumatic engine'. Together with biochemistry and molecular biology, this seems on the point of discovering the secret of life itself.

When we look back and consider how this knowledge has grown we see that successive philosophical systems have played no positive role in it. They have led to no scientific discovery and have usually impeded it, for systems have become dogmas opposed to change, often violently so. The application of scientific method has led to the enlargement of knowledge by accumulating verifiable facts, not by the exercise of abstract reason. To the extent that such scientific experiment abstracts a small part of human experience, comprising certain specifically defined conditions with which certain facts are always associated, the relationship of conditions and facts being demonstrable by anybody repeating the experiment at any time, it represents only one way – the scientific way – of looking at a part of nature. It is this method which has enabled men to walk on the surface of the moon and to discover that mongolism is caused by a defect in the chromosomes, and a method which has brought so much of nature within the field of human inquiry needs no philosophical justification. Nor is it time, as a recent Reith lecturer has suggested to 'take seriously and value forms of perception which do not fall within the experimental model . . . to be attentive to our own feelings as sources of data as good as, and in many cases better than, any sources of data presented to us by our present situation'. One of the forms of perception he advocates is 'existential knowing', a feature of that existentialist philosophy which is a product of behaviourism, which regards man as a collection of trained reflexes. While we accept that no thinking, even that of a scientist considering the evidence provided by experiment, is free of bias and preconception, history teaches us that feelings alone do not provide any sort of guide for the pursuit of knowledge, whereas they have often provided the motive power for destructive and obscurant ideologies which have done nothing but harm.

Relating these general observations to the field of medicine we find that here too the intrusion of theories produced by abstract reasoning has been entirely negative and even positively harmful, because, in this field, the doctor acts out the theories on the patient. It was this situation which Molière satirized when he showed the doctors congratulating each other on the fact that although the patient had died, he had died 'according to art'. Similarly, in these days of 'heroic' surgery we hear a surgeon claiming quite seriously that his operation was a complete success, although unfortunately the patient had died.

The doctor does not treat mankind in the abstract, but an individual man or woman with the aim of curing, or at least alleviating his condition. Unlike the scientist in the laboratory, he cannot defer judgement, and even in less urgent cases, having secured every help that can be gained from his colleagues in the laboratory to diagnose the condition, he has to use his informed and trained judgement to resolve an individual problem. In urgent cases he may have no time for any consultation. It is not sufficient for him merely to have the scientific facts; he has to do something about them immediately. What he does and how he does it depends on his skill and competence as well as his knowledge. To this extent medicine is a practical art which uses the findings of science to achieve its ends. Like other practical arts, it is passed on from one generation to the next by personal initiation and instruction. Because experimental medicine, sharing the methods of investigation employed in the natural sciences, has been so successful, there is a tendency to overlook the fact that in its practice medicine can never be entirely scientific.

An attempt has been made, over the last fifty years in particular, to make the training of the doctor as scientific as possible, cramming more and more of the medical sciences into his curriculum. But it is generally acknowledged that the pace of advance in these sciences is now so great that within a few years of his qualifying as a doctor the information he acquired in the medical school is no longer valid. Since it seems difficult, or even impossible, to provide for him frequent and extended refresher courses, we have to accept the fact that practice must always lag behind the knowledge available at any point in time. But medicine is not unique in this and the time-lag is far less than in many other departments of applied science. What the doctor does retain is the scientific mode of thinking and the independent judgement based on his training and experience. It is this necessary emphasis on their individual independence and their impression that this necessity is not sufficiently appreciated by planners and administrators that makes doctors refractory material for the type of organization that flourishes in an 'admass' culture.

This culture has no great integrating philosophy and doctors are representative of the age in which they live. There is no special philosophy of medicine, although there are vestigial philosophical assumptions which are a hangover from the past. The mainspring of medicine is scientific method, which is now being extended to sociology in an attempt to discover solutions to social problems many of which fall within the medical field. Now that we have computers which are able to programme themselves and therefore 'learn' from experience, it may be that in the coming decades some unifying and general explanation, to which the term 'philosophy' may be attached, may emerge as the product, not of a single intellect, nor of a single 'man of feeling', but of a group of computers initially programmed with all our unanswered questions and all the relevant data to supply the answers.

6

Medicine and Education

In its broadest sense, Medicine is an important department of knowledge; in its narrowest, it is the practice of an art, one of what used to be called 'the useful arts', or applied sciences, now usually grouped under the term 'technology'. Within the present century, although some older practitioners still like to regard their complex of skills and special kinds of knowledge as an 'art', it has become more popular to imply that it is a science, or rather a group of sciences, sometimes called the life-sciences, the bio-medical sciences, or the health sciences. This predilection is certainly a tribute to the increasing scientific precision with which the treatment of disease and the preservation of health may now be understood. At the same time, because up-to-date scientific knowledge (perhaps only temporarily) is more highly regarded than long clinical experience, this choice of view may represent an attempt to make us believe that Medicine, certainly more scientific now than it ever was, is now entirely scientific.

A prerequisite of any medical training is a basic knowledge of at least some of the many sciences which are employed in the practice of medicine, and since this knowledge has to be acquired at a comparatively early age the time given to arts subjects, which many educationists regard as essential to the development of the 'whole person', is necessarily sacrificed. This early bias given to the education of future doctors places them on the side of the scientists in the great division which is said to split our contemporary culture. Whether this schism really exists is a matter of debate, but it is true that the aims and methods of science are frequently misunderstood or brought into question by those without any scientific training. That the principles and practice of Medicine should be the subject of careful scrutiny and challenge is all to the good, for there is a tendency for any specialist to lose sight of the wider aim in pursuit of his more narrow objectives. That there should be actual misunderstanding of the scientists' aims, based on ignorance or distorted information, is likely to prove an obstacle to achievements which are socially desirable. How the ignorant may be taught and how information offered to the public may be better balanced might well emerge from a process of inquiry and research. At the moment all the weight is on the side of scientific novelty, often brought before millions of people in a glamorized form before proof of its ultimate validity has been demonstrated by long use and experience. Every doctor has experience of the patient suggesting or even demanding some new cure or treatment which, scientifically, is still in the trial stage, but which has already been given sensational headlines in the popular press. The expectations aroused by such 'news' are often disappointed. Particular new remedies are found by experience to be effective only in certain cases; or unforeseen side-effects and accidents are recorded; or the organisms regarded as the immediate causes of disease are seen to acquire a resistance to the drug. When these situations occur, there is a natural reaction among the ill-informed so that they turn against well tried and proven scientific treatments and revert to popular remedies of the past. These attitudes are not confined to the ill-educated, for some of the greatest supporters and believers in unscientific treatments have been men and women of high intellectual ability, but usually without much scientific knowledge.

In this chapter we therefore have to discuss two parallel

problems: the education of the doctor and the ways of giving his patients a better understanding of the doctor's outlook and the problems which confront him.

The Education of the Doctor

The aims and methods of medical education are today the subject of constant discussion and criticism, as they have been for well over a century. On the whole the medical profession, in Britain, as in most countries, is very conservative, with a great regard for its traditions and its historic institutions. In the period of rapid social change through which we are passing, doctors are often called upon to defend age-old practices and modes of thought which have themselves helped in shaping the British pattern of medical education. This pattern is essentially an old one, although in the last fifty years much has been done to modify it after a great deal of inquiry and consultation.

For most people, the type of doctor most familiar to them is the general practitioner. But in fact he represents only a minority of all those who receive a medical education and who become registered medical practitioners. The others become specialist consultants, administrators, laboratory workers engaged in medical research, medical officers in the armed forces, employees of the pharmaceutical industry, medical journalists, and so on. All receive the same basic type of medical education before branching out into the special department of medical work in which they make their career.

Medical schools are now part of a university and medical students are undergraduates, but this is a modern phenomenon as far as the majority of the profession is concerned. For hundreds of years the only universities in England were those at Oxford and Cambridge, where medical studies won little academic esteem and were orientated towards theoretical learning rather than to practical ability. When the College of

Physicians was founded in London by Henry VIII in 1518 his chief object was to secure the co-operation of the profession in regulating the practice of medicine so that the lives of his subjects might not be endangered by ignorant and illiterate quacks. Membership of the College was limited to Oxford and Cambridge graduates representing the highest order of the profession and for long they exercised vigorously the disciplinary powers entrusted to them. The College was not, however, a teaching body. It had supervisory powers over the Company of Barber-Surgeons, founded with a royal charter in 1540 and, later, the Society of Apothecaries, a royal foundation of 1617. The three groups – physicians, surgeons, and apothecaries – reflected the strict hierarchy of professional status. Restricted by the terms of their charter to the treatment of wounds, injuries and 'outward' manifestations of disease, the barber-surgeons gradually encroached on the practice reserved for the physicians, as did the apothecaries after them. Originally a dispenser of prescriptions supplied by the physician, by the eighteenth century the apothecary was in effect the equivalent of the modern general practitioner. Few, if any, of the surgeons or apothecaries attended university. They learned their craft by regular apprenticeship, usually begun at the age of 14.

Meanwhile, for want of opportunities for clinical study in Oxford or Cambridge, students of those universities, having acquired the degree of Bachelor of Arts, an essential preliminary, went to the Continent to enrol as medical students in universities such as Padua and Leyden, where medical teaching was of a high order. In the eighteenth century they also came in considerable number to enrol as hospital pupils in the London hospitals, especially St Thomas's and St Bartholomew's. Here they were the private pupils (i.e. apprentices) of the consultant physicians and surgeons, differing only from their humbler fellow-apprentices elsewhere in that their masters were among the leaders of the profession and had the most fashionable and most lucrative practices of their day. With the foundation in the eighteenth century of a number of new hospitals – Guy's, Westminster, the London, St George's and the Middlesex – the attractions of London as a centre of medical education became even more obvious. As the number of pupils increased, their instruction was organized into classes, such as those in anatomy and physiology given by William Cheselden at St Thomas's, and eventually into private medical schools attached to the hospitals but not officially part of them. Although the services which consultants gave to the hospitals, which were all voluntary or charity hospitals, were unpaid, the appointments were eagerly sought after as a means of obtaining reputation and pupils, whose accumulated tuition fees were quite substantial and who remained attached to their teacher, seeking his advice as a consultant when they in turn took up medical practice.

The first such school to give a really comprehensive medical education was the London Hospital Medical College, founded in 1786. The lay governors of the hospital at first complained of the number of pupils whose presence, they thought, interfered with the treatment of patients, but their usefulness as unpaid medical auxiliaries soon became apparent and the complaints were withdrawn. Armed with the certificates of attendance at all the required courses, the students could then present themselves for the M.D. at one of the universities. Examinations were usually perfunctory and oral, with the exception of one, Edinburgh University, where a new medical faculty had been founded in 1726 based on the Leyden pattern. This school rapidly won a high reputation and by mid-century its fame was greater than that of its model. Here came young men from the British colonies in North America who, after gaining the Edinburgh M.D., took home with them the lessons they had learned and established on the same lines in

Philadelphia the first medical school in the United States. Edinburgh graduates also came down to London and presented a formidable challenge to the London doctors and to the licensing regulations which the Royal College of Physicians still attempted to enforce. Making their way to the top by sheer merit, they also proved to be excellent teachers and several of the private schools were of their creation, the most famous being the Windmill Street School of Anatomy where instruction was given by John and William Hunter.

In contrast to Edinburgh, at another Scottish University, St Andrew's (founded in 1411), candidates were not even required to attend in person, it being sufficient to send letters testimonial from two physicians who knew the candidate and were willing to certify his proficiency. The first St Andrew's M.D. was the physician to Queen Anne, John Arbuthnot, friend of Pope and Swift and creator of the character of 'John Bull', while among later recipients was the celebrated Edward Jenner, the pioneer of vaccination.

From the middle of the century onwards a new law permitted anybody who had served in the armed forces in a medical capacity to set up in civilian practice without further examination or licence. During the Napoleonic Wars, the number of young men who had served for a time in the army or navy and then begun practice at home was greatly increased. This fact, added to the ease with which medical qualifications could be acquired, led to agitation for reform. Competition was keen and it was difficult for the ordinary public to tell good doctors from bad. The reformers argued that a licence for medical practice should be granted only to those who had received a regular training and possessed proofs of their competency. In 1815 a new Bill was approved by Parliament which gave the Society of Apothecaries in London the right to examine and license general practitioners throughout the country.

This 'Apothecaries Act', as it was called, was the first step in the development of the modern system of medical education in Britain. The regulations drawn up by the Apothecaries for the new qualifications included apprenticeship to a recognized general practitioner for five years, and a period of hospital practice (which came to be called 'walking the wards') supplemented by compulsory attendance at a course of lectures. Taking into account the prevailing dissatisfaction with the universities' methods of examination – the oral question and answer and the disputation of a thesis – which had persisted since the Middle Ages, the Society was among the first to institute a written examination. This was a great success and the private schools, both in London and the provinces, were given a great impetus by the demands of students wishing to take the examinations. New schools were established at Manchester, Birmingham, Sheffield, Leeds, Newcastle, Bristol, Liverpool and Exeter. Local doctors managed to serve as instructors by giving their lectures in the early morning or in the evening, fitting their business practice in between. For the greater part of the nineteenth century the majority of general practitioners in England qualified in this way. This expanding body of young and well trained practitioners became increasingly resentful of the fact that there was still no law in the statute book which prevented untrained quacks from competing with them for practice. Far from being appeased by the Apothecaries Act, the medical reformers found strong additional support from the newly trained doctors. The agitation continued and achieved most of its aims when a new Medical Act was passed in 1858.

The greatest advance achieved by this Act was the establishment of the Medical Register and of a new General Council of Medical Education and Registration. As its original name implied (it is now simply the General Medical Council (G.M.C.)) its chief responsibility lay with the efficient education and subsequent registration of the duly qualified doctor. The Council came under the authority of the Privy Council (and so of government) and it consisted of representatives of the universities, the professional corporations and the crown, while some thirty years later a representative of the British Medical Association, representing the general practitioner, was added. To accord with the social needs of the day and with the still limited nature of medical and scientific knowledge, the aim of medical education was assumed to be to produce a safe and competent general practitioner. Throughout a century of unprecedented advances in scientific knowledge this remained the ruling concept in medical education. In the report of the most recent of many government inquiries into medical education (1965–8, the 'Todd Report') this concept has at last been repudiated as unrealistic. It is replaced by the view that

every doctor who wishes to exercise a substantial measure of independent clinical judgment will be required to have a substantial postgraduate professional training, and that the aim of the undergraduate course should be to produce not a finished doctor but a broadly educated man who can become a doctor by further training.

The Report goes on to state:

We are convinced that undergraduate medical education should be firmly in the hands of a university and that a university degree course should be a requirement for the entry of British students to the medical profession.

This must seem a truism to those unacquainted with the development of university medical education in Britain in the past century. It is worth recalling some of the more important steps in this development. In 1827, at a time when the original clerical foundations of Oxford and Cambridge still required entrants to accept the 39 Articles of the Church of

England, a group of followers of Jeremy Bentham, led by
Lord Brougham, founded the University of London, mainly
for the higher education of nonconformists. Its chief emphasis
was to be on science and medicine, to which nonconformists
had made important contributions. A new hospital, the
North London Hospital, later renamed University College
Hospital, was founded to give the students clinical instruction.
In 1828 the Church party founded King's College to hold the
balance against what they called 'the godless institution in
Gower Street' and consequently the university was forced to
change its name to University College, both colleges becoming part of the University, which was not responsible for
teaching but only for examining all students before awarding
degrees. The other medical schools in London eventually took
advantage of this special feature, as did the provincial schools.
These latter merged with new Colleges of Arts and Science
later in the century and eventually became the universities of
Manchester, Liverpool, Birmingham, and so on, so that in the
provinces the university degrees in medicine and surgery became the standard qualification, as they were in Scotland. In
London, however, which was the stronghold of the professional corporations, their powerful influence maintained their
own qualifications as the favoured route to entry to the profession. The schools attached to the various teaching hospitals
also maintained closer links with the royal colleges than with
the university, of which they became part only after 1900.
When an American expert on medical education, Abraham
Flexner, inspected the London medical schools in 1912, he
found the bedside teaching excellent, university control mini-
mal, and the general spirit of the schools, especially in the
teaching of scientific subjects, casual and amateurish. He much
preferred the highly organized German system, based entirely
on the universities, as it was elsewhere on the Continent. This
preference was reflected in the recommendations of the Hal-

dane Commission, which in its report quoted Sir William Osler to the effect that

a professor of medicine requires the organization of a hospital unit, if he is to carry out his threefold duty of curing the sick, studying the problems of disease, and not only training his students in the technique of their art, but giving them university instruction in the science of their profession.

War and economic stringency delayed the implementation of these recommendations for many years and it was only with the coming of the National Health Service that the resistance to change shown by the teaching hospitals was eventually broken down. All of them now have professorial units and the university link is now administratively much firmer. Nevertheless, their students remain largely isolated from ordinary university life and so to some extent fail to enjoy some of the advantages which go naturally with a university education. The amalgamation of the schools in pairs to form larger units, as recommended in the Todd Report, will doubtless enlarge purely local loyalties, while their closer linking with the colleges of the university or with new multi-faculty institutions should do much to broaden the outlook of the students.

Following naturally on its recommendation that the undergraduates' medical course shall be only the basic preliminary to advanced training, the Todd Report looks forward to the time when all doctors will be specialists in particular aspects of medicine. This will require an intensive postgraduate training lasting for three years, and when the commissioners examined the facilities for postgraduate education they found them inadequate and haphazard. This is not surprising when we recall that when the Postgraduate Medical School was seeking a home, on its foundation in 1931, none of the teaching hospitals could take it in and it had to be set up in the former workhouse infirmary at Hammersmith. Its reputation is now such that it would add lustre to any of the ancient foundations, but of course its intake is limited and the need is for many more such schools and departments. The British Postgraduate Medical Federation, which had done a great deal in the past twenty years to improve the situation, will certainly find its work and influence greatly increased when the schemes under discussion are implemented.

All these plans depend in the last resort on government finance and government planning. The money will be provided for the schools through the University Grants Commission and for the essential new hospitals through the Department of Social Security. All the planners have to try to forecast the number of doctors that will be required in twenty or thirty years' time and this in turn depends upon likely population growth and upon the advances made meanwhile by existing and possible new preventive measures. We have now, it seems, made up our minds as to what kind of doctor we shall need in the twenty-first century. Whether he will match the needs of the time better than the nineteenth-century model which has had to serve the needs of the twentieth remains to be seen. More important than any precise or accurate prefiguration is the need to ensure that present attitudes do not become fossilized and that plans, institutions, and educational systems have an inbuilt flexibility which will allow changes and improvements to be made at any time without the resistance of traditional vested interests which requires years of investigation and persuasion to overcome.

Many doctors see in the present shifting scene a magnificent opportunity to reshape for the better not only medical education but education in general. It is claimed that the demands of the Health Service introduce an element of consumer control and participation in the training of the doctor which might be taken as a model for education in other vocational subjects, with great benefit, for example, to such careers as those of the engineer and the business manager. The possibilities of co-operation between the universities and industry should be developed on the lines of that existing between the universities and the Health Service. We are reminded that the Royal Society, which is regarded as the Mecca of the 'pure scientist', was founded in the seventeenth century to explore the ways in which science might be used for man's benefit and to increase the prosperity of the country. Intellectual curiosity alone is not sufficient incentive for research, which must always have design and purpose, and means without ends may be, in human terms, meaningless.

It is natural that the universities should seek out as teachers those who have shown themselves able to add to the sum of knowledge by research. Such men and women are not necessarily the best teachers, or if they are they may spare too little time from their research, which can become addictive, for their teaching duties. This conflict of interests is one which is the subject of lively discussion among university teachers today. Although it is not one which greatly affects the teaching of medical undergraduates, it does affect postgraduate education in all the scientific disciplines, including the medical sciences. The personality and success of individual researchers may also have a great influence in the pursuit of certain lines of investigation, both in obtaining financial support and in attracting to it the best brains of particular age groups. The research may not necessarily be that which is best for medicine as a whole, or that which is most urgently needed, but in a free society this is in fact how knowledge advances.

First published in specialist journals, which are the great medium of publication and communication in all the sciences, the new discoveries and new ideas eventually find their way into the text-books which are used by the undergraduate student. The paper in which the new findings are embodied may take nine months or a year to appear. The new edition of

the text-book may be several years later, after years of revision by the author or editor and at least a year in press. It
follows then that at least some of the information contained
in it will need deletions, additions or corrections when the
book is first bought by the student. It is, in short, already out
of date. In a subject where knowledge is growing at such a
rapid pace as it is in medicine, this places a responsibility on the
teachers to ensure that their own knowledge, which has at
least reached the 'journal stage', is employed to advise and
guide the student on new advances. Nevertheless, by the time
he qualifies and begins his compulsory year of hospital service
in medicine and surgery which must precede his full registration (up to that point he is registered as a student) his newly
acquired knowledge is already requiring constant rethinking
and modification. Thenceforward, with the growing demand
of hospital or general practice, it becomes more and more
difficult to keep up, and after five years he should, according
to some authorities, have a refresher course.

Little official notice was taken of this particular education
gap until a few years ago, when postgraduate centres were
opened in many provincial towns. Even now its significance is
not fully appreciated, but if we remember that many doctors
now practising 'finished' their medical education before the
therapeutic revolution began and have had no opportunity
since of even a six-months' refresher course, the size of the
problem can be imagined. It is true that doctors have their
journals and professional societies and that they are profes-
sionally addicted to talking 'shop' on every occasion, but not
all doctors read their journals and not all attend society meetings. While it is also true that the doctor is a perpetual student,
for he is always learning, and not least from his patients, many
would like to see the organization of formal and intensive
study courses, attendance at which should be required at
intervals of say five years.

Nevertheless, even if the doctor manages to keep fairly well abreast of scientific knowledge, he will become increasingly aware, in the course of his work, of the fact that its benefits are not being fully drawn upon. The gap between knowledge and performance remains. The social and economic difficulties responsible for this must be understood if they are to be overcome, and if the doctor, who is also a citizen and a taxpayer and in a special position to see the effects of social health policies, is to help in doing this there is little in his present formal education to prepare him for it. All over the world the signs are increasing that the next stage in medical development is towards preventive and environmental medicine. Medicine is becoming more and more concerned with sociology and if doctors are to discuss problems of community health with social scientists on their own level, or even be able to ask them the right questions, then somewhere in their medical education room must be found for a study of social history and social planning.

Professor Douglas Hubble, who thinks of medicine as a 'humanistic technology', supports proposals made by Sir Eric Ashby for improving the general education of scientists and chooses from them five courses which he, as a medical teacher, considers suitable for medical students. They are ethics, psychology, sociology and social anthropology, the history of technology (medicine), and linguistics and communication. This is an admirable choice, but unfortunately not all medical teachers are as enlightened as Professor Hubble. For many years the General Medical Council has been urging upon medical schools the desirability of reforming and liberalizing the curriculum and some interesting experiments are being made as a result, but many schools are still failing to meet the challenge of the times.

Medicine in General Education

For every doctor working in medicine there are four or five auxiliaries – nurses, physiotherapists, and so on – whose own medical knowledge, on a general, specialist or technical level, must be acquired through training and experience. Outside this immediate circle there are many others to whom some knowledge of medicine is essential or desirable in their work and which they obtain from special courses. But for the population as a whole such knowledge as they have is what they pick up from the mass media of communication, especially television. If this is to appeal to the masses it must never be dull and even while it instructs it must also entertain. Doctors themselves have organized and taken part in many excellent programmes, both for the public generally and in refresher courses for general practitioners, but the requirements of the medium lead to the choice of topics which are sensational and unusual. This would not matter so much if the majority of the viewing public had enough elementary knowledge or understanding of the whole field to see these topics in the right perspective.

The basis of this understanding should be given in primary and secondary education. A little elementary anatomy and hygiene is not at all sufficient for citizens of a world where science and technology supply the dynamic and where the achievements and potentialities of scientific medicine are so important for their future welfare. In earlier times, when medicine was much simpler than it is today, it formed an integral part of everybody's general knowledge. There were 'divers honest persons', to quote the terms of Henry VIII's Act of 1542, 'as well men as women, whom God endowed with the knowledge of the nature, kind and operation of certain herbs, roots and waters, and the using and ministering of them to such as be pained with customable disease'. For centuries the lady of the manor, with her carefully collected recipes and remedies, acted as the unpaid general practitioner for the village folk around, while her husband bought and read with interest and profit many medical books to place on the shelves of his own library.

During the past century medicine has acquired its own special language, which is the language of science and not readily understood by those without any scientific education. The barriers of what irritated arts men have called 'scientific jargon' proved too formidable and medicine dropped altogether from general education as soon as education became compulsory. It is now thought to be one of the subjects which lies on the science side of the abyss which divides the 'two cultures'. In reality, of course, the content of medicine is such that it provides the perfect bridge between them. There are doctors who are poets, painters and novelists, but apart from a few social scientists who have bravely blazed a trail into the field of medical care, there are few who venture in the other direction. The difficulties are great, but not insuperable, and they are diminishing as science teaching improves in the schools and a new generation for whom scientific wonders are everyday matters come into the world to take up their share of running its affairs. Children who are able to digest some of the intricacies of space travel are unlikely to balk at learning much more than is offered them at present about their own bodies, about the nature of disease and health and about the work of the doctor in the community. Teachers are interested and many are anxious to introduce more of these topics into the classroom. But who is to teach the teachers? Suitable books are few and suitable courses non-existent. For many years some teachers of biology and history have been aware of the fact that the history of medicine, showing the contribution which it has made to our present knowledge and to shaping the world we live in, forms a nucleus around which to develop the teaching of elementary medical facts. Text-books representing this kind of approach are growing in number but are still uneven in quality.

The obstacles to the broadening of general education in this way are the present requirements for university entry which force schoolchildren to master a great amount of factual scientific detail if they intend to study any branch of science for their first degree. It has frequently been pointed out that this is demanded by the university teachers themselves, so pushing back the break between the arts and sciences to schooling for the fourteen-year-old. This demand, and the constant tyranny of examinations are distorting our whole educational system. More general scientific studies, combined with arts and social studies are required both in the schools and at the undergraduate level. The men and women of today and tomorrow *must* have a general understanding of science as the key to understanding the world they live in. They do not all have to be scientists.

If such a programme can help the younger generation, it cannot do much to help the older members of the community, except that children always discuss their newly acquired knowledge in the home. Many attempts are made, with more or less success, through many agencies, to inform and instruct the public in medical matters. The doctors' own association, the British Medical Association, which publishes a journal that is read all over the world, founded many years ago a journal for the non-medical entitled *Family Doctor*, as well as many useful booklets on important aspects of healthy living. Hundreds of thousands of copies of these are bought and read, mainly by women who are wives and mothers, the traditional custodians of the family's health.

The Central Council of Health Education was founded in 1927 as a result of a clause in the Public Health Act of 1925 permitting any local authority or County Council 'to arrange for the publication within their area of information on questions relating to health or disease, and for the delivery of lectures and the display of pictures in which such subjects are dealt with, and may defray the whole or a portion of the expenses incurred for any of the purposes of the section.' Strongly supported by the Society of Medical Officers of Health, and with a direct grant from the Ministry, the new Council published journals and year-books and organized meetings, lectures and exhibitions which have had a perceptible influence on the level of health education generally, especially in the work of preventive medicine carried out by local authorities. Its various immunization campaigns have secured the public co-operation in an effort which has all but wiped out the infectious diseases of childhood – diphtheria, whooping cough, poliomyelitis, and it has also sponsored much useful health education in the schools. Now financed entirely by local authorities, the Council should take on added importance – and receive greater financial support – as more government attention is given to preventive medicine. The methods which have proved so useful in the past should be developed and adapted for much larger audiences. The persuasive techniques of television advertising, already familiar to millions, might well be employed on the state system, not just occasionally, but regularly, to convey information which is so vital for the health and welfare of all.

7

Medicine and Politics

THE government of every civilized country has to make some provision for safeguarding the health of its people. Even at a minimum, the protective measures of communal hygiene, including sewage disposal, the supply of pure water, the compulsory notification of infectious diseases, the inspection of industrial premises and places of public resort, the licensing and regulation of medical practitioners, all demand expenditure of public money and the state's employment of medical personnel in an executive or administrative capacity. Nor is government concern with health limited to a department of health, for practically every aspect of government has some influence on it, through education, housing, town-planning, industry and trade, and particularly social security, with which the department of health in Britain is now linked.

Today it seems an essential and obvious responsibility of government, and it is one which at once brings medicine into the political arena, not only on a national but on an international scale, for disease knows no frontiers. Practically nonexistent in 1800, except in special emergencies such as epidemics or wars, it was by 1900 a recognized part of the normal functions of government, although it had not yet achieved the relatively high status it is given today. In part this transformation has been effected by the scientific advances made in medicine, in part by the growth of democracy and by political movements which place the opportunities for a healthy life among the forefront of the rights of the people. The spread of universal education and the information propagated by the modern mass media have also acted to make people everywhere aware of the elementary necessities for a healthy life and of what can be done to prevent disease and to treat illness when it occurs. In our own time too, the wealth which has been expended on two world wars has made everybody conscious of what it is within the capacity of a united effort to achieve. Comparisons have been made between the money spent on wars or preparation for wars and what is spent on some of the basic necessities. It has been suggested that a cure for cancer would already be known if the same time, thought and money had been devoted to it as is given to the space programme of either the United States or the Soviet Union. The order of priorities has been set by political decisions and a change in that order will have to be achieved by the same means.

There are political parties in many countries which are pledged to this aim, that is, to reduce expenditure on such traditionally costly items as defence and to spend more on hospitals, housing and schools. The campaigns to achieve these ends are often conceived in black and white terms which tend to present more cautious planners of public expenditure as heartless oppressors of the poor. But this oversimplifies the problem. In the long run, to take a simple example, it may be of greater benefit to the national health to improve an existing road system and so cut down the number of serious injuries and deaths from accidents than to build a great new permanent hospital which the advances of medicine may make structurally obsolete before the end of its useful life, or which policies of education and professional training may make it difficult to staff adequately.

If we study the development of government responsibility for health matters in Britain we find that it was exactly a century between the establishment of the first General Board of

Health in 1848 and the beginning of the National Health Service in 1948. The Board was set up when the country was expecting its second epidemic of cholera and after the publication of Edwin Chadwick's classic report on the sanitary condition of the labouring classes. It lasted only six years, falling victim to the monumental unpopularity of Chadwick and his plans for sanitary reform. The hostility which he aroused may be imagined when we read one of the most celebrated passages of his report:

Such is the absence of civic economy in some of our towns that their condition in respect to cleanliness is almost as bad as that of an encamped horde, or an undisciplined soldiery. . . . The discipline of the army has advanced beyond the economy of the towns. . . . The towns, whose population never change their encampments have no such care, and whilst the houses, streets, courts, lanes and streams are polluted and rendered pestilential, the civic officers have generally contented themselves with the most barbarous expedients or sit still amongst the pollution, with the resignation of Turkish fatalists under the supposed destiny of the prevalent ignorance, sloth and filth.

He considered that the medical profession gave him little or no help in his struggle and that the current medical controversies on the causes of fever diverted attention from the practical means of prevention of disease. He saw the chief remedies for the appalling situation presented in his report as 'applications of the science of engineering, of which the medical men know nothing; and to gain powers for their applications, and deal with local rights which stand in the way of practical improvements, some jurisprudence is necessary of which the engineers know nothing.' For him 'the great preventives were drainage, street and house cleaning by means of supplies of water and improved sewerage, and especially the introduction of cheaper and more efficient modes of removing all noxious refuse from the towns. . . . For these operations aid must be sought from the science of the Civil Engineer, not from the physician, who has done his work when he has pointed out the disease that results from the neglect of proper administrative measures, and he has alleviated the sufferings of the victims.'

It took the country some time to recover from Chadwick's shock treatment. He was sacked, albeit with a handsome pension, at the age of 54, but time has its revenges and he would have rejoiced to see the day when a British government was to include a Minister for the Environment. His work was taken up, with a tact and diplomatic skill which Chadwick totally lacked, by Sir John Simon, who was appointed to a new post, that of Medical Officer to the Privy Council, and later, in 1871, to the new Local Government Board. The fact that he was a medical man who had done great things as the first Medical Officer of Health to the city of London appeased the medical profession and for twenty years his quiet and pervasive influence on government helped to bring about many of the reforms demanded by Chadwick as well as considerable reforms in the organization of the medical profession itself.

The last three decades of the nineteenth century were occupied with the consolidation of the achievements of the reformers so that by 1900 a whole new field of activity for central and local government had been created.

Many of the matters now included under public health were delegated to local government and financed from local rates. The very fact that they were charged with these important duties gave a great impetus to the newly fashioned and reformed local authorities. Even ratepayers came to realize that the best councils were not necessarily those that spent least and that the revenue from local taxation could be well invested in community welfare from which all benefited. Particular cities and towns took a pride in their local services and often went beyond the national government in correcting particular evils as they became obvious. The Education Act of 1870 also brought them new responsibility and further enlarged the sphere of their activities and eventually, when the Schools Medical Service was begun in 1908, the Schools Medical Officer joined the Medical Officer of Health in guarding the health of the community. Maternity and infant welfare clinics, and special out-patient clinics and long-stay sanitoria for those suffering from tuberculosis also came within their province, as well as isolation hospitals for other infectious diseases such as scarlet fever, smallpox and diphtheria. All these activities were supervised by the Local Government Board, a branch of central government which in 1919 became the Ministry of Health.

The second achievement of government in the medical sphere was to regulate medical practice so that a qualified and well-trained medical profession was available for the treatment of disease. Some halting steps had been made in this direction three centuries earlier. The first Medical Act was passed in February 1512 to protect the king's subjects against hordes of quacks and impostors who were preying on their credulity and ignorance. There was no nationwide system of local government at that time and the only authority with adequate powers to control medical practice was the Church. The bishops were therefore authorized to license good and honest practitioners whose respectability was vouched for by their neighbours and whose skill was confirmed by a panel of two or three qualified doctors or surgeons. Continuing the Tudor reformation of government and administration, Henry VIII gave a charter for the foundation of the College of Physicians in 1518 and another to the Barber-Surgeons in 1540. But both were much too small to provide skilled and licensed medical care to all and in an Act of 1542, which came to be known as 'the Quacks' Charter', the king, charging the surgeons with 'minding only their own lucres', exempted from the penalties laid down for unlicensed practice 'divers honest persons, as well men as women, whom God hath endowed with the knowledge of the nature, kind and operation of certain herbs, roots and waters, and the using and ministering of them to such as be pained with customable diseases.'

This Tudor legislation clarified by subsequent celebrated cases in the courts, remained the basis of government control of medical practice until the nineteenth century. The only addition was the granting by James I of a charter for the incorporation of the Apothecaries in 1617. Originally concerned only with the dispensing of the medicines prepared by the physicians, the apothecary soon became the 'poor man's doctor' and, by the nineteenth century, the general practitioner. Controversy between the three branches of the profession was perennial, the two 'lower orders' constantly fighting off attempts by the physicians to enforce their legal rights of control. At the beginning of the last century, as a product of the ferment produced by the French Revolution and the Napoleonic wars, some kind of concordat was reached. A new College of Surgeons was granted a royal charter in 1800. A pressure group of medical reformers, largely made up of apothecaries, had some measure of success when the Apothecaries Act was passed in 1815, with the concurrence of the College of Physicians. This Act entrusted to the Apothecaries the major responsibility for training, examining and licensing the general practitioner and was most successful, so successful indeed that the increasing numbers of regularly trained doctors came more and more to resent the active competition of those who had undergone little training and no examination. The 1815 Act therefore did not still the demands for reform but gave them a new stimulus. After decades of planning and agitation the Medical Act of 1858 established the General Medical Council and the Medical Register. It did not appease the doctors by making unqualified practice illegal, but preserved certain rights – the signing of death certificates, medical appointments under the state and so on – to qualified and registered medical practitioners.

Three years earlier, in 1855, the Provincial Medical and Surgical Association, founded by Sir Charles Hastings nearly twenty-five years before, became the British Medical Association. This was purely a professional body, with no legal control over medical practitioners and, for thirty years, no representation on the General Medical Council to which this control was entrusted. Throughout the first century of its existence the Council (generally known as the G.M.C.) did much to raise the standards of both general and medical education in the profession and was particularly successful (through its Disciplinary Committee) in eradicating most of the objectionable and unethical aspects of medical practice as it had been known for centuries. The B.M.A. was more concerned with assuring and improving the status of the profession *vis-à-vis* the state. It fought bitterly the introduction of the first National Health Insurance Act in 1911, when Lloyd George, rather belatedly in fact, wanted to lay a firm basis for the medical care of the lower-paid workers by state insurance, something which had already been well established in Germany.

And here we come to the third sphere where government has accepted responsibility – the provision of medical care for the sick. At first it was only the sick poor, and in certain times and places only sick paupers, who could benefit from this provision. Under the Elizabethan Poor Law of 1601 it was usual for a parish to secure the services of a doctor by the payment of an agreed annual sum, often little more than £20 or £30 a year. The sick poor within the parish were then treated as required by the doctor without further expense to the parish. When the Poor Law was amended in 1834 the new

Commissioners, who were given no specific guidance on medical treatment in the Act, expressed concern at the fact that in many parishes medical relief was given to all the labouring poor and not restricted to those who were technically paupers. In accordance with the deterrent principles on which the new legislation was based, the recipients of indoor or outdoor parish medical relief were now required to be labelled as paupers. In practice, it was rare for such relief to be denied to the respectable poor who were in need because of illness rather than improvidence. In the manufacturing and mining towns of the north, some medical care was provided either by employers or through dispensaries, friendly societies and medical clubs organized and maintained by the subscriptions of the workers. This kind of 'club practice' survived into the present century and became much disliked by the medical profession because of the low salaries and the great demands made upon the doctor's services. The committees of workmen who ran such clubs were often found to be even worse employers than some of the Boards of Guardians.

The provision of this 'cut-price' medical care was only possible because the doctor was simultaneously in a position to make his living from private practice and his services to parish or club were regarded in much the same light as his gratuitous service to the local voluntary hospital. It was possible only as long as it did not make such demands on his time and energies that insufficient time was left for private practice. At its inception, the National Health Insurance Act of 1911 was a new departure only in the centralization under government of a great many independent provident and insurance schemes. Like these, the new Health Insurance covered only the breadwinner earning less than £160 a year, the wife and children still requiring paid medical treatment when they were sick. For serious illness the voluntary hospitals were available for both classes of patient, some contribution to costs being made by friendly societies or hospital savings associations.

The political storm in which the government became involved with the doctors when Lloyd George announced his plans has been described as the worst in which the medical profession in Britain ever took part. It was certainly marked by far more bitterness among the doctors than was ever aroused by the plans for the National Health Service a generation later. Since the working of the scheme would affect for the most part the general practitioners in the poorer quarters of industrial towns and cities the B.M.A. rather than the royal colleges led the attack on the government's plans. With their experience of 'contract practice' and their treatment by friendly societies and clubs, the general practitioners feared they would become enmeshed in one vast 'contract practice' for the workers where doctors would be overworked and underpaid. They also resented the control of the medical service by laymen. However, Lloyd George steered a conciliatory course with his usual skill and eventually won the day by agreeing that health committees on which the doctors themselves would be represented were to control the new service. When the Secretary of the B.M.A. with the approval of his Council, accepted the office of Vice-Chairman of the National Insurance Commissioners, many B.M.A. members saw themselves as betrayed by their own Council. But their battle was already lost in the country, where public opinion was against them, and in Parliament, where the overwhelming strength of the Liberal Party was available to see the Act implemented with all possible speed. In the event, it proved successful as far as it went, covering about one half of the workers in the country. It was the first step in the campaign to establish a system of medical care for all the people, a campaign which gathered strength between the wars, in a period of great unemployment and depression, and then reached the stage of practical planning during the Second World War.

When the Bill was introduced in 1946 it was the product of several years of discussions between government and the medical profession together with social welfare and other agencies. Despite this, there was again an outcry from the doctors about the terms of the service, but as before the political leaders knew that the country was strongly behind them and that the hospital service, which had not been covered by the Act of 1911, had been rescued from bankruptcy only by the establishment of the Emergency Medical Service at the outbreak of war and could not continue without massive state aid.

It is only in the last century that hospitals have become places where the majority of people expect to be treated when they are ill. In Victorian England, the sick poor often regarded the journey to hospital as 'the last ride' and admission to hospital as a death sentence – this in spite of the fact that statistics reveal that a substantial proportion of all patients admitted were in fact treated successfully and discharged cured. Nevertheless, that prejudice reflects the grim aspect of the hospitals of those days, where the patient was always conscious of being an object of charity in an institution where the hazards of ill-informed and unskilful treatment were matched only by those of cross-infection and exceeded only by those existing in the insanitary and overcrowded dwellings of the poor. The transformation to what we know today has been achieved by the phenomenal growth of the medical sciences and a corresponding increase in the skill, knowledge and scientific aids available for both diagnosis and treatment, all of which are now concentrated in the hospital. Simultaneously, there has been a great improvement in the conditions of what the Victorians called 'the labouring classes'. Much better educated and informed, they are more keenly aware of medical possibilities than could have been even guessed at by a doctor of an earlier age and believe that if a condition *can* be cured then it *must* be cured, or somebody is at fault. They demand and expect the best possible treatment when they are sick and this usually implies treatment in hospital, either as in-patient or out-patient.

This being so, no Health Service that called itself 'National' could possibly have been established which did not bring in all the hospitals, so that it was readily accepted by all concerned that they should be nationalized. In July 1948, when this great undertaking was started, the government became the monopoly supplier of all medical care in the country. Although private practice was still permitted it could not really compete to an extent that affected the situation. Some of the private insurance schemes have persisted and some have prospered by a judicious mixture of state and private expenditure. There are 'pay-beds' and private wings in state hospitals which offer some patients the chance of more privacy and some amenities not available in public wards. But it must be emphasized that the professional care given to patients is the same in both sectors. The existence of what has been called 'first and second class' medical care is attacked by some who do not fully realize that their implicit comparison with railway or air travel is not so harmful as they intend, for a train or an airplane is handled with the same experience and skill for all its passengers and all have the same chance of a safe arrival. If some prefer to spend a great deal more upon the extra comforts available and thereby reduce the pressure upon space elsewhere, this is surely one of the individual rights which need not be sacrificed.

That there are considerable differences in medical care in various parts of the service cannot be denied, but there are both geographical and historical factors which account for these. Despite an ambitious hospital building programme, long deferred because of economic difficulties, most hospitals in the service are relics of the past, comprising in their number former poor law hospitals (workhouse infirmaries), municipal hospitals, small charity hospitals and cottage hospitals. The difficulties of staffing all hospitals adequately at a time when skilled medical and nursing personnel is in short supply are too well known to need discussion. It would be idle to pretend that the same types of skill, knowledge and equipment are available in all kinds of hospital, but the speed of modern transport helps to overcome some of these deficiencies by the transferring of acute and difficult cases to specialist departments of larger hospitals where more may be done for them. The great London teaching hospitals, all of which were once charity hospitals, have few staffing difficulties because of their reputation rather than the modernity of their buildings, some of which are little better than the old infirmaries. It is possible that more might have been done in the past twenty-five years if doctors had not kept their sights fixed so firmly on the monumental type of hospital which was the ideal of a past age. The local authorities and charitable bodies which built or rebuilt so many hospitals in the second half of the nineteenth century at a time when labour was cheap, opened with great pride the very buildings which we find so troublesome and expensive to maintain today. A general extension of the use made of temporary single-storey hospitals by the wartime Emergency Medical Service would have made it possible to abandon these obsolete and insanitary structures which have provided material for so many complaints against the Health Service.

Nevertheless, the majority of people are satisfied with the National Health Service, and if fewer doctors are now enthusiastic about it their disappointment or disillusion springs from the periods of economic stringency which have perennially dashed their hopes and laid upon them the necessity to continue working in conditions which are far from perfect. Successive Ministers of Health have been aware of this dissatisfaction and inevitably they have borne the blame for the persistence of these conditions. They reply, quite reasonably, that the funds available are not limitless and that it would never be possible to do more than bring about a gradual amelioration until eventually all the older hospital buildings are replaced. As for the present staffing difficulties and the undoubted exploitation of younger hospital doctors, these are the direct result of a political decision taken by a former government acting on the recommendations of the Willink report on the training of doctors. This report concluded, erroneously as it turned out, that too many doctors would be trained in Britain unless the medical schools cut down their intake. The error is now acknowledged and steps are being taken to reverse the trend.

It is a well-known fact that the National Health Service would be in danger of a complete breakdown if it were not for the many thousands of doctors and nurses from former British colonies who are now employed in the hospitals. At the same time the country loses several hundreds of British born doctors each year by emigration, a large proportion of them to the United States. The irony of this situation is brought home to us if we look at the medical needs and services of the countries – the developing countries – from which they come. Trained in British style medical schools established in the days of dependency they come hopefully to Britain for postgraduate training. Too often, unfortunately, they become just 'another pair of hands' caught up in the necessities of the time and their routine duties make it difficult for them to get through the studies necessary for their higher qualification. When they do succeed and return to their own countries they find in the cities a great number of similarly trained and qualified doctors who have trodden the path before them and are now competing for jobs in urban communities which, by British standards, are already over-doctored. In India, for example, about 20 per cent of the population enjoys the services of nearly 90 per cent of the doctors, the ratio being one doctor to less than 1,000 patients. The remaining 80 per cent of the people, living in a rural environment, have little more than 10 per cent of the doctors, about one doctor to 43,000 people. Their medical training has made the doctors feel that it is impossible to employ their professional skills without the suitably equipped hospitals in which these skills have been developed. A cardiologist who has received his advanced training in Britain or the United States, accustomed as he will be to resuscitation units and monitoring services for acute cardiac emergencies, may well feel it impossible to carry on his work in an Indian village community or even in a town with a hospital with little modern equipment. Sooner or later he is likely to swell the numbers of those seeking a career elsewhere.

An illuminating example has recently been cited from Thailand, where American advisers asked to consider the problem of the great concentration of qualified medical personnel in Bangkok recommended that a new medical school should be opened in a provincial city and so develop a second medical centre. This was done, the school being designed and run on American lines. The first class of medical graduates from this school lost no time after qualifying in chartering a plane and emigrating en bloc to the United States. If the question immediately springs to mind, 'Who is helping whom?' we do not cast doubt upon the motives of all such aid schemes, but upon the planning which contributes high level medical specialists to a people which really needs village doctors and health visitors.

But the supply of doctors is only one facet of a very complex problem which is encountered everywhere in the developing countries. Basically, the peoples in these countries lack the organized and comprehensive system of public health common in the developed countries and without it the communicable diseases are still practically unchecked. Sanitation and water supplies are the fundamentals for a safe environment in cities and with population increase the systems laid down in the late nineteenth century by colonial governments have long since proved utterly inadequate. Overcrowded cities in tropical regions present the same kind of threat to health as the industrial populations of mid-nineteenth century Britain protested against and one or other of them may yet become a focus of infection which may assume epidemic or even pandemic form. The cost of remedying this situation grows from year to year and reaches formidable proportions when compared with the resources available to particular governments.

Most of these countries are agricultural, but crop failures and occasional famines are only the more sensational symptoms of a larger failure in government planning and organization of food resources. Combined with a persistent failure to provide more than a slight elementary education to a small proportion of the people, which in turn makes all plans for health education difficult if not impossible, these factors reinforce the disparity between the Western type medical graduates and the field where their labours are needed. Here, indeed, a political transformation is necessary before any medical problems can really be solved.

If we return to the developed countries, we find that Britain is not alone in the difficulties of providing medical care to all its people. Other European countries also suffer from a shortage of doctors, notably Italy where, as to some extent in Britain, the middle class families which once supplied the professions no longer find sufficient prestige or rewards in the practice of medicine to attract their sons. Unlike Britain, however, their places are not being filled by recruits from a lower social level and in fine old medical schools such as Bologna there is more than enough room for native students so that vacant places are filled by students from abroad. In the United States, Medicine is still one of the most rewarding and prestigious professions, so that ten applicants may be found for every place in a good medical school. It so happens that New York State recognizes the M.D. degree of Bologna and many hundreds of young American doctors have first graduated at Bologna and successfully presented themselves at the State Boards in New York State for the licence to practise. In many countries, again unlike Britain, where medical students are notable for their absence from political demonstrations and other expressions of student unrest, the medical schools are suffering, with other departments of universities, from the current wave of disorders and demands for reform of academic organization. What effect this will eventually have on medical education and the kind of doctor produced by the medical schools remains to be seen.

Some standardization of training and licensing throughout Europe seems almost inevitable as a result of an enlarged Common Market and eventually, some kind of federated or united states of Europe. With common recognition of qualifications and mutual arrangements for medical care of patients other than natives the possible mobility of trained doctors and nurses will be much enlarged and so introduce new strains in the working of our own National Health Service.

Meanwhile, in the United States, where the systems of medical care current in Europe are often regarded and referred to as 'socialized medicine', there must remain for some time a gap in medical manpower which foreign medical graduates will inevitably fill. A recent report by the Carnegie Foundation puts the present number at about 46,000 or 15 per cent of the total and calls for a 50 per cent increase in the annual production of trained native doctors. This report is extremely critical of the present system of medical care in the United States and especially of the private insurance schemes which in fact cover only a little more than 20 per cent of the total costs. Despite this, and despite the fact that it proposes an immediate doubling of federal funds for medical education, the report has not been rejected by the American Medical Association, but is described as 'consistent with the Association's feelings and beliefs' and as 'timely and useful'. It seems therefore that opinion is veering towards at least some measure of 'socialized medicine' even in the stronghold of private enterprise.

The significance of such trends may be taken as indicating the fruition of a generation's efforts to encourage attitudes of social responsibility and is a healthy sign. Now medical science is adding its weight to the pressures exerted by an uneasy social conscience, for, as the American report emphasizes, many new discoveries and treatments are not being made available to patients through the existing system. We have seen the choice of medical care systems pushed into the centre of the political scene, but as the basic framework becomes accepted everywhere as a government responsibility it will, to that extent, be taken out of politics and become the subject of operational research to rationalize and improve delivery. It is unthinkable that any political party could, or would wish to, 'denationalize' the Health Service in Britain, but without some solution to our economic problems, its weaknesses may take some time to remedy. With the speed of change that is customary in the United States it is even possible that a federal service may be established there which will far outstrip the British model. Even in Europe, recent statistics make it clear that the service which was once a courageous experiment and a model for the world is now lagging behind what is being done elsewhere.

Some critics of the Service suggest that it should be 'taken out of politics' and by this they mean that it should be removed from direct government control and established as an independent corporation like the Post Office or the B.B.C., with a large proportion of professional staffing and responsibility. This proposal would be more realistic if the Health Service was actually paid for by insurance contributions, but the majority of the expenditure comes from general taxation and no government could consent to handing over an annual expenditure approaching £500m. to any kind of independent organization.

This is only one of many proposals to find a way out of current dilemmas, another being the suggestion that responsibility for health care should be delegated to local authorities. These bodies already receive large sums from central government for general education and are already responsible for public health services within their areas. But here again, the vast sums involved would make it impossible for government to delegate responsibility for expenditure of this order and any such move would be against all present trends.

The present regional boards, with their various committees, already give a substantial amount of local representation. The boards themselves, the members of which give voluntary service, are appointed by the Minister for a set term, but the board is entirely responsible for selecting the members of the hospital management committees and for supervising the administration of the service within the region. With some half a million employees throughout the country, each board is responsible for the activities of about 50,000 people, and any business concern of comparable size could only be managed successfully by tight budgetary control and some machinery for continuous examination of the results of all its various operations. With no profit and loss account to crystallize its results, the Health Service can only be judged by consumer satisfaction, and where the consumers are in fact the whole people then any Minister, and any government, must take account of their wishes.

Despite this, the Service still lacks any central body which is fully engaged on operational research into the service. Most ministers have found, like Chadwick, that the medical profession does not speak with one voice. Highly trained to make individual decisions, doctors often differ in their opinions of what should be done on any specific occasion, but the Minister has to seek lay advice and to carry the country with him so that whatever he decides, some doctors inevitably think him wrong. The kind of operational research which would produce facts instead of opinions and offer guidance to a Minister on objective grounds is a great desideratum.

Scientific medical research is of course one of the major activities which comes within the responsibility of the Minister and on which a great deal is spent. This began as part of government sponsored work in the time when Sir John Simon was developing the Medical Department of the Privy Council a little over a century ago. Although its significance and importance was not fully understood by the politicians they eventually allowed a small expenditure under pressure from the medical staff. When the National Insurance Act was passed in 1911 the government of the day promised to add one penny to the contribution paid by every individual worker covered by the scheme in order to finance the work of a Medical Research Committee, later to become the Medical Research Council. Beginning with an annual budget of about £50,000, the Council now has nearly £20m. a year, its research headquarters being established in a National Institute of Medical Research at Mill Hill, with numerous other research laboratories for specific problems located in universities and hospitals throughout the country. Its pattern of research is based mainly on the laboratory, but its fine series of Special Reports include classic investigations of tuberculosis, nutrition, pneumoconiosis and other medical problems of great social importance.

The national expenditure on medical research also includes

financial support provided through the University Grants Committee to individuals and departments working in universities and from philanthropic bodies such as the Nuffield Foundation and the Wellcome Trust. To this must be added the research carried on in the private laboratories of the pharmaceutical industry. From the point of view of curative medicine this has been most productive over the last thirty years and has resulted in the introduction of many new drugs for the treatment of human and animal diseases. The pharmaceutical industry has been the subject of many political attacks based on the size of the drug bill in the National Health Service, but these attacks overlook the high cost of the research factor in every new drug. Two-thirds of the production of the industry are exported and the prices charged are necessarily those which are current in the world market. To balance the cost of drugs, which represent less than 10 per cent of the cost of the hospital service, we must also put in the scale the saving on expensive hospital treatment by avoiding admission to hospital altogether or by reducing the length of stay of those admitted.

Twenty years' experience of the Health Service and of public and private argument on its operation has underlined the weaknesses which were enforced at the time of its inception by the compromise between several opposing interests. Fear of a full-time salaried service in which doctors would be 'civil servants' under the direct control of politicians led to the compromise whereby general practitioners remain theoretically in the position of individual private contractors to the service who are also able to carry on private practice, if it is available. Hospital doctors are employees of the service, but at the consultant level they contract for a certain number of sessions (half-days) each week, may engage in private consultant practice elsewhere and are also eligible for 'merit awards', substantial annual bonuses graded in amount according to the status and achievements of the individual consultant. The Medical Officer of Health and other medical and paramedical staff of local authorities remained as direct employees of the local authority on fixed salary scales.

This situation reflects the tripartite structure of the service with little or no machinery for integrating it. General practitioners, who used to staff many of the smaller hospitals, so that they could follow through a case, no longer had access to hospital beds and complained that they were reduced in status to form-fillers whose chief task lay in referring their patients to hospitals. Because few practitioners had available the kind of scientific equipment now considered essential to accurate diagnosis, a referral to hospital became the customary first line of approach and the normal expectation of patients suffering from more than minor ailments. In his discussion with doctors at the beginning of the Service Aneurin Bevan had promised that 'health centres' would be established where groups of general practitioners would be able to share diagnostic aids, secretarial services, and the collaboration of social workers, health visitors, and nurses who were already part of the local authority staff. In such a centre the practitioner would be a member of a closely organized team which could do much to promote the health of the local population. Because of economic difficulties and for other reasons a succession of governments were slow to implement this promise and only in the last few years have the centres begun to be provided in any number. Meanwhile the general practitioners have established their own Royal College as a counterweight to the consultants in the Royal College of Physicians and in recent years have been far less concerned about their public image. All present trends are towards a much more closely integrated health service with the main burden being shifted away from the understaffed out-patient departments of the hospitals to the local health centre. There should also be much more opportunity for genuine preventive medicine and health education so that the service really becomes a National Health Service and not, as it has been called, a national disease service.

Fortunately, when we look at the international scene, it is the peaceful and orderly development of the modern local authority preventive service rather than the controversial National Health Service which has provided the model. Soon after the turn of the century the Pan American Sanitary Organization was set up in Washington to deal with international sanitary regulations and quarantine as they affected the American continent. In 1907 an International Office of Public Hygiene with twelve member states was established in Paris to study and report on these matters throughout the world. When the League of Nations was formed after the First World War, it set up its own Health Organization at Geneva which soon outstripped the old International Office in the usefulness of its work for world health. It published a weekly bulletin of epidemiological information and made special studies of the world prevalence of malaria, plague, tuberculosis, trypanosomiasis, cancer and heart disease. International committees working under its auspices gave valuable guidance on the nomenclature of diseases, with particular reference to the classification of causes of death (an essential preliminary to accurate statistics of morbidity), on housing and rural hygiene and in 1935 it issued an important report on nutrition.

Its successor is the World Health Organization, which now represents 130 member states. Established on 7 April 1948 after discussions lasting two years between the states forming the new United Nations Organization, WHO (as it is commonly referred to) is the executive arm of the World Health Assembly with headquarters in Geneva and regional offices in Copenhagen, Brazzaville, New Delhi, Manila, and Washington. Financed by contributions from its member states (of which the United States pays 31 per cent) it has been singularly free from political argument or dissension. It took over all the problems which had been studied by the former international body and has made substantial and positive progress with several of them, its most ambitious programme being its project to eradicate malaria in countries where it had long been endemic. In addition it has developed continuing programmes of great importance concerned with maternal and child health, venereal disease, parasitic and virus diseases, mental health and environmental sanitation, as well as with hospital and public health administration. Its greatest direct beneficiaries have been the developing countries and in an attempt to aid these countries in the urgent problems arising from the 'population explosion' it set up in 1965 a Human Reproduction Unit to research and advise on contraceptive programmes.

The value of such an international body as WHO – and of its parallel United Nations creation, the Food and Agriculture Organization – cannot be estimated only by the immediate results of its activities in solving world health problems. The experience of wide cooperation in health care is a useful basis for similar joint action in other spheres. The countries represented and involved in it have all to some extent a stake in its eventual success which they would not easily abandon and it may well be that Medicine, which has certainly benefited from political action and political decisions, will eventually transcend politics and itself modify political behaviour.

8

Medicine and Economics

FOR the individual living in a welfare state a serious illness is not the personal catastrophe it once was. He knows that his dependants will not starve or lose their home because of his sudden loss of earning capacity and that all the medical care necessary to restore him to health will be provided without charge. For the breadwinner living in a country where medical care is regarded as a 'consumer good', to be bought and paid for at the point of consumption, his illness alone can have disastrous effects on the way of life and future expectations of his family. Most countries in the world have a system of health care more like the first than the second of these extremes. Even in the United States, where the second has long been defended, it seems only a matter of time before the economic 'realists' have to give way to the demands of the majority that is most likely to suffer under the present system.

The defects of this system have recently been revealed in a report issued by the Carnegie Foundation* which shows that the medical advances made over the last twenty years are not being applied to all patients. Many Americans receive care of a very poor quality or none at all and in infant mortality and life expectancy the United States is far behind other industrialized countries. The private health insurance schemes, which are supposed to cover almost the entire cost of illness, in practice cover only 22 per cent of the patient's total costs and exclude

* *Higher Education and the Nation's Health*, McGraw-Hill, October, 1970.

all out-patient treatment. Doctors are highly trained medical specialists and the standards in the best hospitals are the highest in the world, but all medical staffs are over-worked (with an average of 60 hours a week) as a result of a chronic shortage of physicians, nurses and technicians. The cost of medical care is constantly rising and in 1968-9 the collective cost was over $60,000 million, or 7 per cent of the gross national product, a higher proportion than that expended in the welfare state.

Recent opinion polls have shown that a majority of Americans feel that they are not getting value for money and that medical care is overpriced and its organization inefficient. They would like to see an extension of Medicare, the system recently introduced to cover the medical needs of retired workers, to cover the whole working population. Even the American Medical Association, which has bitterly opposed any form of what it calls 'socialized medicine', accepts the criticisms found in the Carnegie report and supports its recommendations.

Before coming nearer home to discuss our own National Health Service, it is worth glancing at the way some other European countries tackle this problem. Germany had the first compulsory health insurance scheme, established in 1883 by Bismarck's government. At first under 'consumer control', like the many contract schemes for club doctors in the industrial areas of Britain at that time, it was very unpopular with doctors, who secured a transfer of control to the Insurance Doctors' Association in the first decade of this century. This Association now acts as the agent for the insurance bodies in each *Land* in distributing remuneration to individual doctors from a central pool. Payment to doctors is not on a capitation basis but is determined by the services given, these being priced according to an agreed tariff. The central pool in each *Land* is not a fixed amount but is negotiated regularly at short intervals, taking account of the number of inhabitants and their average income. Patients make no contribution to the cost of treatment. Critics of this system declare that it is open to abuse by both doctors and patients and that it is expensive and complicated to administer.

In France, on the other hand, a scheme which was established in 1930 requires the patient to pay the total fee direct to the doctor (except for in-patient treatment, when the hospital is paid direct by the insurance body), and then to claim a refund of 80 per cent from the insurance body. In practice, this refund has never amounted to so large a proportion of the fee, for the doctors have always complained that the official tariffs were too low and they came to an 'understanding' with the patient whereby he is paid at a much higher rate while the patient's refund is calculated on the official valuation of the services rendered. Sweden has a similar scheme and although the refund (75 per cent) is lower, it does bear a closer relation to the amount which the patient actually pays out. Denmark's scheme is almost as old as Germany's, but it has no central pool of remuneration. The doctor has a choice between payment by capitation or by item of service, the former being preferred in most towns while the latter is chosen by most country doctors. In the Soviet Union and in Israel there is a full-time salaried medical service.

In Britain, when discussions were proceeding preparatory to the introduction of the National Health Service, one of the possible features was the establishment of a full-time salaried medical service. This was strongly opposed by the British Medical Association at the time as it was feared that the central authority would have too much power over clinicians and interfere with the doctor-patient relationship. It was also realized that the State would be a monopoly employer and so be in a position to dictate terms. Although a considerable number of doctors, even clinicians of various kinds were even then salaried employees of local authorities, some of which had full-time consultant physicians on the staffs of their hospitals, there was little evidence that the doctor-patient relationship had indeed suffered. Indeed, with the cash element removed from individual consultations many doctors felt less inhibited in recommending what they thought to be medically justified rather than what was economically feasible for the individual patient.

In the event, the service was a compromise. The method of paying general practitioners already familiar under the National Insurance Act of 1911, that is, by a capitation fee, was continued, so allowing them if they so wished, to continue in private practice as an addition to their insurance work. All hospital staffs are paid on a salary basis, with consultants having a choice between full and part-time service according to the number of sessions attended each week, based on a notional total of eleven sessions (or half-days). Consultants also receive additional remuneration in the form of merit awards, graded according to their status and experience, the top award having the effect of doubling their basic full-time salary.

After nearly twenty years' experience of the service, it became clear that it was threatened with deterioration through manpower shortage and inadequacies and anomalies in the structure of remuneration. The Review Body on Doctors' and Dentists' Remuneration, set up by government in March 1962 under the chairmanship of Lord Kindersley, made detailed recommendations for an entirely new pay structure which came into effect in 1967. These particularly affected general practitioners. The old central pool, limited to a predetermined amount and then shared between practitioners, was abolished, and instead of a simple capitation fee and practice expenses, a basic practice allowance is paid to all principals in a practice with at least 1,000 patients with service available at normal hours within certain minimum periods each week. Additional allowances are made for group practice, since investigation had shown that this was something to be encouraged, and for stand-by duty at nights and at week-ends. The standard capitation fee is continued for each patient, but the fee is increased for patients over 65. Doctors willing to accept duties outside normal hours are paid a supplementary capitation fee for each patient on their books above the basic figure of 1,000 and also a separate fee for each visit actually paid between midnight and 7 a.m.

The effect of this new system has been to halt the drift away from general practice and to regenerate this section of the profession. Expense allowances up to 70 per cent of the cost of ancillary help have helped to remove one of the greatest causes of discontent, the burden placed on the doctor's wife who often acted as unpaid secretarial assistant. The discontents within the hospital section of the service were more demonstrably centred on the junior hospital doctors and were attracting popular attention through the activities of a new Junior Hospital Doctors' Association. The limitation on the number of consultants employed in the service made for an unprogressive career structure.

Because they wish to be specialists rather than general practitioners, young qualified doctors seek posts in the hospital service after they have spent the compulsory postgraduate year as house officer. Here, as senior house officers, junior and senior registrars in succession they may pass more than ten years becoming highly skilled in the hope that they will eventually obtain a post as consultant. It has been calculated that, with the comparatively low salaries they are paid, their own personal investment, in loss of earnings that they could have made over this period in general practice, amounts to more than £25,000. The earnings of consultants are now much lower than they once were and may never repay the individual for the earlier sacrifice. The workload is heaviest on this section of the medical staff of a hospital and the shortage of manpower is such that study periods and study leave, essential for preparing for the higher examinations which qualify for consultant status, cannot often be taken. This situation led to the so-called 'brain-drain', with hundreds of highly trained young doctors emigrating each year to the United States and other countries. To remedy its own manpower shortage the United States employs nearly 50,000 doctors (or 15 per cent of its total) from foreign graduates, paying them more than double (in real terms) what they could earn at home. The State has itself invested many thousands of pounds in their training and can ill afford to lose them.

By increasing salary scales throughout the hospital service, but with a larger proportional increase in the salaries of junior doctors, the Review Body eased the immediate pressure on the service to some extent. Since 1967 plans for new medical schools have been put in train and existing schools have increased their intake. With the post-war bulge in the birth-rate now flattening out and a larger age-group moving out of childhood years when more demands are made for medical care, it seems likely that some long-standing problems in the health service may cease to exist. The progress of the hospital building plan, whereby new district hospitals are taking the place of a number of obsolete buildings, expensive in maintenance and manpower, will further ease the situation. The growing number of health centres with group practices and ancillary aids should take some of the workload off the hospitals, which have been used far too much for routine tests and examinations and for trivial complaints. On the other hand, the rate of inflation and rising costs in the last year or two threatens to make remuneration once more a point at issue between government and the profession. In 1970 the Labour government rejected a further series of recommendations of the Review Body, and its chairman resigned in protest. The declared intention of the same government to abolish the independent Review Board and to entrust the Prices and Income Board with periodical reviews of professional remuneration was followed by its own fall from power and the abolition by the succeeding Conservative government of the Prices and Income Board itself.

A former Minister of Health, Mr Enoch Powell, once said that a new Minister on appointment may soon get the impression that all he will ever be able to discuss with the professional bodies representing the doctors is remuneration. It is indeed true that it seems to lie at the root of many of the problems encountered in the service. As a profession, doctors depended for centuries upon the fees paid them by private patients and their earnings and standard of living varied as greatly as their status. Some doctors, especially those who were physicians or surgeons to the great and the wealthy, had very rich rewards, but they served without payment as honorary consultants in charity hospitals. Many doctors of the middle rank also secured incomes which ranked them with lawyers and other professional men, and they too often charged very little, or nothing at all, for treating the poor. But many doctors also made little more than a modest livelihood from their practice and were anxious to supplement it by accepting an annual blanket fee of as little as £50 to care for the sick in a workhouse infirmary or to supply medical services, as required, to the members of a trade union or friendly society, or medical club based on a local industry. The 'panel system' set up by the National Insurance Act of 1911 at least ensured that they got something for treating sick workers who could not afford to pay and saved them a considerable burden of bad debts which would eventually have to be written off.

Under the National Health Service the various grades of the profession have drawn closer together from the point of view of remuneration. No doctor in Britain today could earn anything like some of the incomes made by distinguished consultants in late Victorian England, but no doctor could be as poor as some of those working in the industrial slums of the same period. Improved education and training has also made the profession more homogeneous. Arguing from an existing basis of private practice in 1946, the British Medical Association was moved by the fears of its members that a state salary structure might remove opportunities of earning incomes far larger than could be provided under any state scheme.

It was not realized at the time how complete would be the transfer of the fee-paying middle-class patients to treatment under the health service. At first tentatively, and then enthusiastically, the great majority of such patients tried out the benefits of the service and appreciated the value of what they received. The result was a rapid fall in the amount of private practice, and even with the growth of private insurance schemes, to which individuals contribute almost entirely for hospital care in pay-beds or private wings of state hospitals, it is now only a very small proportion of general practice and many young doctors today have no experience of it. At the present time the majority of all doctors on the medical register are in receipt of salaries, for the number of general practitioners, on whose behalf the rather complicated pay structure of the 1967 scheme was evolved, total fewer than 25,000. Despite the general resistance to change in the profession, it seems possible that after the present scheme has been operating for a period long enough to provide standards for a salary scheme, a proposal may well be made for this to be reconsidered.

Perhaps the greatest obstacle to it is the fact that the representative bodies of the profession are regularly forced to engage in public (and highly publicized) debates about their remuneration, for want of any provision by which scales could be adjusted upwards to guard against inflation and to preserve relative rewards in real terms. This is of course common practice in trade unions, but by taking part in it a professional body may well feel that its public image is tarnished. It is also a fact that public service employees are often the last to obtain a revision of scales when economic circumstances demand it. The unfortunate economic difficulties through which Britain has passed in the last twenty years has exaggerated this tendency, but given a stable economy, with even a modest, if regular, rate of growth, it should not be impossible to devise a system whereby agreed standards could be automatically maintained and improved as conditions permitted.

Although doctors' pay, like the cost of drugs, has been a perennial source of friction in the health service, it must be remembered that these are items, and not major items in the annual cost of the health service. In the year 1969–70 this amounted to £1,704·5 million, of which the hospital service accounted for £1,166·7 million while all general practitioner services totalled £147·7 million gross, or £127·8 million net. When the service was set up many people wrongly believed that it was to be paid for by the health insurance contributions. It is not. In 1969–70 the revenue from this source amounted only to £180·3 million, only little more than 10 per cent of the total cost, the remainder being met almost entirely from general taxation. The total cost has risen steadily from £968·8 million in 1963–4, with £661·2 million on the hospital service, to the present figure.

But medical care is only one, if the most obvious, of the services which must be financed to assure the health of the people. Over the whole field of preventive medicine there is also government and local authority expenditure, to which must be added the money spent by nationalized and private industry in connection with occupational diseases or other hazards to health. The education and training of doctors, nurses and other paramedical personnel, with all the necessary capital investment in buildings and equipment, as well as medical research, represent a further charge on public funds. Certain items which appear under other heads on the national budget are also more or less clearly related to the health of the people. Outstanding among these are social security, housing and slum clearance, the improvement of public utilities, education and schools. Together with the health services, these items account for about one-half of all the revenues raised by taxation. Sickness absence, with temporary or permanent incapacity and premature death among the employed population, with consequent loss of productivity, must also be included in the total cost of ill health and this, judging from average earnings, amounts to approximately £1,000 million a year.

It may be recalled that in his famous report Lord Beveridge anticipated an annual cost of about one-tenth of the present figure at the beginning of the service and that the cost would decline rather than increase. This assumption was based on the belief that with a reduction of disease resulting from the activities of the health service the demand for medical care would be correspondingly reduced. While it is true that many infectious diseases have been practically abolished or remarkably reduced in incidence, other diseases have increased to take their place. People are certainly living longer and so becoming more subject to diseases which take a long time to develop, such as lung cancer and heart disease, which are now major killers. The proportion of the population who are over 65 years of age and retired from active employment has also greatly increased and, together with young children, make the greatest demands on the service.

The trend throughout the world is for expenditure on all aspects of welfare to rise and international comparisons show that expenditure in Britain, substantial as it is, is in real terms declining. The cost of medical care is bound to rise yet further.

Advances in the sciences, whether it be in biochemistry or nuclear physics, have their effect on medicine. New methods of diagnosis, new treatments, techniques and apparatus are developed and as soon as they become available they create a demand which must be met, however expensive they may be. Theoretically, there is no limit to the amount which may be spent. No country in the world is rich enough to allocate unlimited resources for this purpose. This being so, it follows that, unless the Conservative Government in Britain transfers a substantial section of the health service to a separate insurance scheme, an attempt must be made to ensure that better use is made of existing resources within a fixed budget.

The possibility of doing so would be greatly improved if more were known about the actual operation of the service. With a budget approaching £2,000 million and employees numbering more than 600,000 the service has no central information and planning body. Despite all the individual reports on separate aspects of the service which have occupied many thousands of man hours devoted to them by distinguished members of committees, the need is still for an operational research unit which would consider all these aspects and their relationship to each other and to the end product, the delivery of medical care. Something well staffed like a government institute of health economics (and business management) would be necessary to maintain a constant scrutiny of all the factors involved and to recommend changes as they became necessary.

Failing such an impartial and scientific investigation on a continuing basis we shall have to go on depending on the research and arguments of rival economic theorists, politically aligned one way or the other, on *ad hoc* committees whose reports may be shelved, and on the alternative schemes presented by directly interested bodies. One such is a report on *Health Services Financing*, commissioned by the British Medical

Association in 1967 and published in May 1970. The brief for the Advisory Panel responsible for this report was 'the urgent preparation of an alternative health service in which financial provision would be less dependent upon taxation'. Like the work of many recent committees, it was overtaken by events in that the Labour Government decided on an administrative reorganization of the health service which would remedy an initial weakness of the service by integrating hospital, general practitioner and local authority medical care. Nevertheless, it is claimed that these changes do not affect the main financial arguments. On the assumption that the service is inadequate and will become increasingly inadequate because of insufficient finance, it suggests that the only way out of the *impasse* is to divide the service into two sections, one which would continue to be financed by taxation and a second which would be financed by a separate health insurance scheme. The first would comprise all local authority and pharmaceutical services (the 'drug bill'), all expenditure on administration, education and research, all capital hospital expenditure, and all recurrent hospital expenditure on the chronic sick, the aged and the mentally subnormal. The second would account for all other expenditure which would be met by a compulsory insurance scheme designed to meet the economic cost of the services rendered. This would apply to the whole population, but those receiving an income below a certain figure would have their premium subsidized. Medical care available under the scheme would be basic and to some extent limited, but those who wished to insure for something more than the 'utility' standard might contract out of the basic scheme and insure under a more expensive scheme which would presumably offer the same kind of facilities as are now offered by BUPA and other private insurance schemes. Payment would be made to the hospital, general practitioner, dentist or optician by the insurance body on a fee for service basis, item by item.

The reception of these proposals, which are still being discussed by B.M.A. members, was, predictably, coloured by the political and social outlook of the commentators. Some saw in it a threat to dismantle the health service, to which Dr Ivor Jones, the chairman of the Panel, replied that the Panel had 'stated its belief that it was neither desirable nor practicable to think in terms of dismantling the health service. Indeed, the members . . . accepted Mr Kenneth Robinson's definition of purpose in the foreword to the first Green Paper: "The paramount requirement is that all the different kinds of treatment that an individual may need at different times, whether separately or in combination, should be readily available to him."' The proposal to develop a system which offered first and second class medical care also came under attack, to which the chairman's reply was:

Acceptance of the principles upon which this system has been based must result in an increased allocation of national income to the health services. The only sacrifice that would have to be made would be the concept of equality within the National Health Service. But this objective has not been realized at any time and never could be. Choice must lie between the illusion of equality in underfinanced health services provided from general taxation and a system such as that proposed, which, while deliberately allowing variations in standards of medical care, raises the standard of such care for everyone.

Some critics of the plan, while allowing that the service would not cease to be 'national' if its financial basis were changed from 90 per cent taxation and 10 per cent insurance to 50 per cent of each, question the possibility of allowing 'variations in the standards of medical care'. It is argued that it is a doctor's ethical duty to restore a patient to health by all means possible and as soon as possible regardless of cost, and that treatment itself leaves no openings for deliberate variations from this desirable aim. What is left are incidental amenities – private beds and/or rooms and such 'extras' as go with them. But do these justify the introduction of a two-tier insurance scheme? It is presumed that all who desire these extras are already contributing to the £50 million a year which is spent on private medical care, yet the report anticipates ten times this sum from the same source, and it would probably require more. Arguing from the fact that £25,000 million is spent each year on consumer goods, the report suggests that a small percentage of this sum diverted to paying for medical care would be enough to ensure the stability of the health service. The problem is discussed in terms of the 'market' and consumer choice, it being suggested that many people would prefer to pay more for their own or their family's medical care than is at present spent by the government. The critics retort that illness itself is not a matter of choice, like the purchase of a new car, but comes unexpectedly, out of the blue, and that the consumer is not qualified to judge the quality or standard of the medical care for which he would be paying.

It is recognized that the chief difficulty in service financing springs from the drift in the national economy and the fact that Britain is spending a smaller proportion of its national income on medical care than most other developed countries. The report's financial projections show that the rate at which expenditure on the service has grown over the past ten years cannot be sustained without (a) an economic growth rate of 4 per cent or more a year (as against the present 2½ per cent), (b) an increase in taxation (which the present government has promised to reduce), (c) a rearrangement of priorities on expenditure on the social services (which would leave other welfare services starved of finance), or (d) budgeting for a deficit. Since none of these accord with government economic policy then the health service, if no fresh source of revenue is opened up, will necessarily deteriorate. This analysis has not been challenged and the present government, with its election promise to leave more of his own money in the pocket of every elector still ringing in its ears, is faced with the dilemma for which this report offers one possible solution. It seems unlikely that the service will see the end of its first twenty-five years without crisis and radical change, for it is in the interest of neither doctors nor patients to allow the kind of drift into stagnation of which overworked staffs, closed wards, and casualty departments restricted to business hours are only the first symptoms.

Although it may seem parochial in a general discussion of this kind to give a disproportionate amount of space to the British health service, the fact that it was the first comprehensive national service made it a social and technological experiment which has been closely watched in many other parts of the world, not least in America. Its very existence has certainly had a great influence on the provision of medical care elsewhere and it may now have to borrow features which have proved successful in other schemes in order to overcome its present difficulties.

But there are other aspects of medicine and economics which should not be forgotten. Among these are the possibilities of reducing the incidence of disease and disability by a more positive approach to preventive medicine. A specialist (P. W. Bothwell, see bibliography) writing on this subject has suggested that the soaring costs of medical care might have been avoided if a greater investment had been made in preventive medicine at the outset of the health service. He argues that a great deal of expenditure is incurred in treating disease which, at only a fraction of the cost, might have been prevented by research and health education. Mass screening for tuberculosis, diabetes and cervical cancer has already succeeded in revealing disease at an early stage when prompt action can be taken and before a long, disabling and perhaps fatal illness has to be given medical care. Fluoridation of water supplies, still inadequately applied because of ill-informed opposition in some regions, prevents dental caries among children and saves a considerable expenditure on dental care. The proper use of the services, especially the local authority services such as maternity and child welfare clinics, needs to be brought home to those who need them most, the poorer and less well educated classes. The connection between social class and infant mortality is well established, but too little is done to redress the balance. The greatest proportion of accidents which are brought to the casualty department are those which have occurred in the home – burns, scalds, cuts and fractures – the number of which could be reduced by education, simple precautions (such as fire-guards), or the removal of hazards. Death and injury on the roads have reached epidemic figures, but the rate of increase is already being slowed down by the improvement of 'black spots' on the roads, the building of new roads and motorways, the compulsory use of safety harnesses and crash helmets and improvements in the design of motor vehicles. Publicity campaigns to drive home the dangers of cigarette smoking, especially among children and young people, would cost only a fraction of the cost of lung cancer. A positive and enlightened programme of family planning would not only reduce the abortion lists but would reduce the load on the health and welfare services in connection with 'one parent families'. It would also be an appropriate contribution for a developed country to make towards the solution of the world population problem.

Publications such as the B.M.A.'s journal *Family Doctor* and the topical booklets regularly produced under its aegis are a valuable addition to the media of health education. They are bought and read mostly by women but not usually by women in the social classes most in need of information and advice. These would certainly be reached by a sustained and well organized campaign on television, where the professional approach and expert assessment of results found in independent advertising of consumer goods might well be employed. There is available in B.B.C. television an opportunity for using all the techniques to which the viewing public are known to respond for the benefit not only of the nation's health but eventually of its wealth too.

But even wealth brings its health problems. In a world where plenty and poverty coexist even the so-called affluent society may contain substantial segments of its population as poor as many in an underdeveloped country. Even in Britain's welfare state there is much poverty among the elderly. Increasingly segregated from the younger and better-off members of the community, having spent a working life which has seen low wages and long years of depression, hardship and war, they are now condemned to spend their declining years either alone or in institutions restricted to members of their own age-group. Tax and pension systems are so arranged as to exclude them from normal employment at an age when many are still active and healthy and still anxious to contribute what they can, even in a different way, to the national economy. For want of such opportunity, through boredom, loneliness and undernutrition, they become ill, at first with trivial ailments, and eventually add to the numbers filling the geriatric wards of the State hospitals. A more positive and more humane approach to this problem, in the form of a government scheme of re-training and redeployment and changes in the tax and pension schemes, is long overdue.

An affluent society also creates new diseases. Obesity is a result of its own form of malnutrition combined with lack of physical exercise, and coronary heart disease and lung cancer are not serious problems among the poor of Africa or India. New industries and new waste products contribute to the increasing pollution of the environment, which is now seen as one of the growing threats to health in all developed countries.

Moreover, it is a pollution which cannot be restricted to national boundaries. Radioactive dust in the upper air and methyl mercury in the oceans are both mutagenic and may be the cause of developmental defects in children yet unborn. It might well be an appropriate recompense for a fine to be levied on all countries or industries which polluted the environment in this way so that ample funds might be provided to the World Health Organization for research and action to counteract existing dangers and prevent the creation of similar dangers in the future.

The developed countries of the world already contribute aid to the developing countries, but only a small proportion of it is allotted to medical programmes. The British contribution amounted to only 7 per cent of all the aid given by Western countries and it is now an accepted target that every developed country should contribute 1 per cent of its gross national product. Between them, the developed countries spend more than £20,000 million each year on their own public health, which is ten times more than all the money spent for the same purpose in the developing countries and more than twenty times more *per capita*. The ways in which this much smaller amount is being spent in the developing countries are being questioned by some of those more closely concerned with the aid programmes. In particular they question whether the model of Western medicine, with its high rise hospital blocks, research laboratories and 'chromium plated gadgetry' is at all relevant to the needs of the newly independent countries. It is often taken by the governments of those countries as a status symbol, like an independent air line, but is in fact quite uneconomic. The money might be better spent on training a large number of medical auxiliaries who would then be paid incentive salaries to encourage them to work in rural areas where no kind of medical care is at present available. Such auxiliaries would be of great value in furthering maternal and child health by staffing small local clinics and especially by running family planning programmes and contributing generally to health education.

Britain helped to establish and develop medical schools in its former colonies, all on the British pattern, and the successor governments sought British advice in expanding them. These have now produced a great number of good doctors, but all better fitted to practise their profession in a country like Britain than in the agricultural areas of India and Pakistan. More than one-half of all the junior doctors employed in the British health service are now such foreign graduates, educated at the expense of their own governments, whose aid is essential to maintain the British service, just as the aid of British doctors is essential to providing adequate medical care in the United States. When we, in the developed countries, talk of aid to countries less fortunate than ourselves, we should remember that the obligation is mutual and that the aid we give them now is not only a recognition of the benefits we had from them in colonial days but of the benefits which the richer countries are still receiving from the poorer.

All the topics touched upon in this chapter are today the subject of keen debate in many countries. This is in itself a healthy sign and already some of the mistakes that have been made in the past are being corrected. If at times we have the impression that the search for health is a will-of-the-wisp and that no stable balance will ever be achieved, it is salutary to remind ourselves of what has already been achieved and endured. It is now more true than it ever was that 'health is wealth', for ill health is now manifestly so wasteful and expensive that no intelligent government will neglect means of preventing it.

9

Medicine in the World
of Tomorrow

WHEN we look back over the last thirty years and consider all the changes which have been made in the world since 1940 we shall probably agree that although some of the specific changes might have been predicted many of the most important could not have been foreseen. New discoveries in science and technology have transformed the possibilities of providing enough for all and emphasize the fact that it is social and political planning which must now ensure that the means are employed to this end. Although we have gone some way towards this in that aspect of life which most concerns us here – man's physical and mental health – very much more can and will be achieved in the next thirty years.

All forecasts made today, however, must be even more subject to error than any that was made in the past as a result of one unprecedented and inescapable fact. For the first time in his history man has the means to bring about his own destruction and to render the planet which we inhabit incapable of supporting life as we know it. If the shadow of the hydrogen bomb seems to have receded, compared with ten or fifteen years ago, it may be that we are better able to avert our gaze from it, accepting and rationalizing its existence by pointing to the effects of a 'balance of terror' in staving off a war between the major powers. The brief excursions made by medical historians into the political and military history of past world crises, demonstrating as they do the effect of a leader's ill health on crucial decisions, should make us all realize that the world cannot be safe as long as such a weapon is at the disposal of any man, however great he may be considered as a world statesman.

Even the by-products of the bomb, and of other chemical and biological weapons of war, could become a major hazard to world health through the problems of storage and disposal of waste. Rather late in the day, for biologists have been trying to drive home the lesson for twenty years, we are becoming conscious of the importance of a clean environment and beginning to take steps to prevent its pollution. Just as the Victorians were passionately determined to ensure the purity of the water supply to a town or city, so we must determine to prevent the poisoning of the air we breathe. Already in the United States a warning has gone out to manufacturers of the internal combustion engine that legislation to ban its use in cities is on the way and that some other form of powered locomotion must be found.

But this is only the most obvious of many sources of pollution which will be identified and banned in the coming decades. Some kinds of fertilizers and pesticides which are washed from the soil into rivers and eventually into the open sea are also under suspicion, as well as the known chemical poisons in industrial wastes and effluents which are cumulative and which find their way into plants and animals used as food. Even the widespread use of antibiotics and steroids in the food industries must be watched for its possible deleterious effects on the health of man and especially for the role of such use of antibiotics in developing resistant strains of micro-organisms which are harmful to man. The chemicals which are added to food for colouring, flavouring and preserving will also be under constant scrutiny and once any substance is suspect the rapid dissemination of the information will lead to pressure on a government to ban its use. Although these measures are negative, they are all positive steps in removing potential dangers from the human environment which fall legitimately within the province of preventive medicine.

Indeed, we are likely to see very much more attention paid to all the preventive aspects of medicine than has been given to them in the past. It will be seen that this is the best way of making a balanced and effective medical care a practical possibility. The great advances which have been made in curative medicine in the past thirty years have been applied to lessen the burden of disease inherited from the past, but it is only one phase in the long history of medicine. Younger, healthier generations are now being recruited to the working populations of all communities and by the time they reach retiring age it is likely that the medical care of the elderly will pose fewer and less urgent problems than they do today. This is assuming, of course, that many of the psychological stresses associated with advancing technology can be kept within bounds. As long as automation can be made the servant and not the master of man it can release many millions of men and women from tedious and soul-destroying routines of mass production. The right of leisure will become an important contributory factor to mental as well as physical health. Improved educational standards demanded by the new industrial processes will enlarge the interests of many and make possible for them a creative and dynamic instead of a simply passive role in their recreation. The many fine old crafts which are dying out because the machine can make their products more cheaply will find a new and uncommercial value as men and women rediscover the joys of making things with their own hands and in their own time.

Long before the year A.D. 2000 the present barriers to the developing potential of trade and industry – largely artificial barriers of international finance – will be removed, and in a richer world the working populations of the developed countries will have worked off their hunger for the material goods that industry can supply and divert their energies to some of the more abiding and less basic purposes of life. Already the young are seeking some higher purpose than the satisfaction of their immediate appetites and it is probable that this will be found, whether in the creation of a new social order or a new religion remains to be seen. In a period which even some bishops refer to as 'post-Christian' many of the young feel a spiritual hunger which few pretend to satisfy. If they require this to be satisfied in order to feel they are real people living a full life then it seems likely that this need will be met. With such a change in social outlook health would improve dramatically. Apart from a declining curve in the incidence of mental illness, which now accounts for more than half of all illness in developed countries, there would also be a fall in those disorders which are known to have a psychosomatic component. Sickness would no longer, consciously or unconsciously, be used to such an extent as a refuge from personal frustrations and dissatisfactions.

The liberating effect of these changes on doctors themselves would also be beneficial, for nothing is more frustrating to a doctor than treating patients who do not want to get well or who persist in behaviour which is harmful to them and makes further calls on him inevitable. Doctors would themselves receive less of the limelight than they do now, when there is an almost morbid and sensational interest in disease and its treatment. In Plato's ideal republic the presence of many hospitals and doctors in a city was a sign, not of a compassionate society, but of a bad government, and in Butler's *Erewhon* illness was a crime. These are extreme attitudes, of course, but from the biologically long-term view are much more conducive to the future health and welfare of man than the deliberate preservation and fostering – even to the point of breeding – of genetical misfits and defects.

How far we should go in our efforts to guard against any

possible danger to health is not entirely a matter of available money and manpower. Health is a balance of opposing forces and if the balance is destroyed by removing too much weight on one side the cause of health is not served. In the laboratories today the effects of breeding laboratory animals in sterile conditions provide a model of what might happen to the human race if it were ever possible to reproduce these conditions in our immediate environment. Fortunately for those healthy reactions in man's 'interior environment' which are essential to his future protection against disease, it is not possible. Despite the hopes of many visionaries, while disease can be controlled, it can never be abolished, for it is, like death itself, a factor in our human environment. However much we should like to see freedom from illness and from pain as part of the human birthright these are freedoms that can never be guaranteed, but illness and pain are risks that can be minimized as far as is humanly possible.

Here again, the extent to which they should be minimized may have to be decided on scientific rather than emotional grounds. It has been observed that over-protective conditions, in which animals are allowed to satisfy their needs without much conscious effort on their part and from which all possible stresses and frustrations are removed, show glandular and biochemical changes which unfit them for life in the natural state. How to divert rather than suppress the natural aggressive drive of young manhood, how to provide the challenging situations essential to the young man's full and healthy development which will benefit rather than harm the community in which he lives, are problems which are not yet satisfactorily solved. What used to be called 'divine discontent' is a valuable source of social energy and even if it expresses itself at times in violent demonstration it may still be more desirable than the apathy and complacency of others. In a world that has been sated by the violence of unprecedented wars we must not over-react against physical aggression (even in the cause of non-aggression!) by an age group to which it is biologically natural. Our own violence against them may be less physical and more subtle, but far more damaging to society in the long run.

These are not the only ethical problems likely to demand our attention in the world of tomorrow. The 'population explosion' has been described as a greater threat to the future than the existence of the hydrogen bomb itself. In a sense it is linked with it, for the pressure of growing populations in Asia for a greater share of the world's material resources could result in a war in which the bomb might be used. At least one of the 'think-tanks' in the United States has already analysed the probable effects and outlined the measures necessary for the survivors. The other grim prospect associated with this problem is mass starvation. During the past few years the world's population has been growing at the rate of 8 per cent per year while the food resources have been growing at the rate of 5 per cent. Simple arithmetic makes the outcome clear, but in this area some unpredictable discovery may ease the situation. Cheap artificial protein is already being made from the waste products of the oil industry and man's ingenuity and technological capacity may well find other ways of filling the gap.

However, confronted with problems of such magnitude we must indeed despair if responsible leaders of thought and morals have no better response to make than a ban on contraception. Morals are made for man and have changed with changing societies and changing needs. There is nothing absolute or eternal about them. The dignity of man and the sanctity of human life are values which are likely to be better served in stable societies where the quality of life is steadily improved rather than in conditions to which even formerly peaceful animals have reacted by psychotic aggression. Fortunately, both governments and international organizations are alert to the growing danger and the same agencies which have helped to create the problem by applying modern medical discoveries in the developing countries and greatly reducing infant mortality are now following up their work with rural clinics and advisers on contraception. What is needed, however, is a world-wide campaign to eradicate age-old ideas that a large family is a credit to its parents, and to instil the view that it should be taken as a particular mark of social irresponsibility. All voluntary methods will certainly be insufficient and there will be great pressure for all governments to pass laws limiting the size of families, to abolish all incentive schemes such as family allowances and to replace them with positive inducements such as extra tax benefits which will be forfeited when another child is added to a young family. This too will only be applicable in the richer countries, an essential measure to match the egalitarian demands of the day. In those countries where the threat is developing most rapidly compulsory sterilization and/or abortion after the birth of the third child may well become government policy. In the meantime, medicine is making its contribution to a solution by the development of new oral contraceptives. It is confidently predicted – and it is a prediction based on research now going on – that by 1975 fertility control by mass medication will be possible, but it will of course require government action to direct its use. Alternatively, there will by then be available a 'male pill', a pill for taking after intercourse, a long-acting pill, and a technique for immunizing against pregnancy.

At the other end of the life span, the advances of medicine will certainly lead to a healthier and more active old age. At the present time the average expectation of life at the age of 65 has not increased dramatically, for those who survived the hazards of childhood in the first decade of the twentieth century, the two world wars and the economic depression between them, now succumb to the slowly developing diseases which are associated with age. Not only will much more be learned about these diseases and how to prevent and cure them, but each group that enters this last period of their lives will do so with a healthier life history behind them and with increasing prospects of many years of active and healthy life ahead of them. These will not be helpless and apathetic old people to be segregated in homes for the aged but men and women of experience with a positive contribution to make to the family and to society. For them retirement would not be a life of compulsory idleness but a change of activity and many of the good causes that languish at present for want of suitable helpers should benefit. Their increasing numbers will of course add to the population problem and perhaps provoke intensified campaigns for legal euthanasia. Society itself will have to decide the issue and not leave the burden of decision to the doctors whose first duty will be, as it always has been, to preserve and prolong life. An Englishman who is now a saint of the Roman Catholic Church, St Thomas More, considered it a social duty of the old and sick to choose to die, and if our ethical standards have changed since his day they could as easily change again under the pressure of necessity.

If we now leave these general problems and adjust our focus to take in the more specific field of medical and scientific research, we can still only use as a basis what is already known and developing at this moment. Nobody can predict the kind of new discovery, like the antibiotics, which comes out of the blue and sets going a whole generation of researchers on new lines of inquiry. The topics which are occupying more research man-hours than any others at the moment are all types of cancer and heart disease. Considerable progress has been made in the past thirty years in our understanding of these diseases. None of the specialists is at all optimistic that a cancer cure will be found tomorrow – but of course that too may come out of the blue. If it does it is most likely to come from research in cell metabolism and genetics.

The effects of certain carcinogens (cancer-producing substances) on the chemistry of the cell are already being studied and a recent report from the Sloan-Kettering Institute in New York suggests that we shall soon have a clear picture of the way in which certain viruses produce some kinds of tumour. A prolonged study of chemical carcinogens at the Chester–Beatty Institute in London proved that many naturally occurring tar products, some of which are found as combustion products of tobacco, are responsible for others. Now that all the evidence linking smoking and cancer is overwhelming we shall certainly see within the next decade both a revulsion against tobacco which will make smoking socially unacceptable as well as more positive measures by government to control its use. The vast economic interests involved in the growth and use of tobacco are already well aware of this and they will redouble their research efforts to produce a safe product which will satisfy the emotional (and chemical) needs of the consumers. It seems probable that much useful research will also be carried out to discover why many heavy cigarette smokers do not develop cancer.

The search for specific anti-cancer drugs has been going on for some time, but it is a difficult one because of the variety in causation and character of the different types of cancer. It is not a question of destroying a particular invasive organism without harming the surrounding tissues, such as Paul Ehrlich set out to achieve in his search for a 'magic bullet', for with cancer it is the patient's own cells which are responsible for the new growth. When safe anti-cancer drugs are developed – and useful cytotoxic drugs are already in production – it seems inevitable that hopes will be raised that cannot be fulfilled, for it is likely that their action will be limited to one particular type of tumour and to have no effect on others. However, the use of such drugs will provide growing points of knowledge which can then be gradually extended to deal with hitherto incurable types.

From a field which has no immediate connection with cancer – that of organ transplants – other help may come. The new science of immunochemistry initiated by Sir Macfarlane Burnet and Sir Peter Medawar has been rapidly developed to find ways of suppressing the immune response which makes the body reject a transplanted organ. This is one of our most fundamental protections against infection and comes into play when any foreign body (in the form of a transplant) is grafted on to the body. Chemicals have already been developed which suppress this mechanism for a time so effectively that the patient has to be kept in a sterile environment in order to guard him from infection. More specific types of drug will be found which leave much of the protective immunity unimpaired but suppress the particular immune response which is responsible for the rejection. Conversely, for the understanding of this phenomenon is growing so rapidly, other drugs are likely to be found – perhaps almost by accident – which promote rejection, not of a graft, but of a malignant growth, and so make a valuable contribution to the treatment of cancer.

Meanwhile, our present treatment of cancer will continue to improve, and its results should not be under-estimated. Surgery, radiotherapy and appropriate drugs already succeed in arresting many types of cancer, and experts consider that within the next twenty years more than two-thirds of cancer patients will be successfully treated in this way. This proportion may be significantly increased if the new techniques which make possible early diagnosis are more widely used.

We have already mentioned transplant surgery, the possibilities of which received world-wide publicity when Mr Christian Barnard succeeded in transplanting a human heart.

The difficulties associated with this procedure have also been mentioned, and the ways in which they might be overcome. Less publicity has been given to kidney and liver transplants, which may present greater technical problems to the surgeon but which are also finding a useful place in modern surgery. The transplantation of the whole heart may be restricted to certain specified cases now that another operation has been developed in London for replacing the patient's incompetent coronary arteries with veins taken from his own thigh, which are not of course subject to rejection.

These are desperate measures which are employed only after coronary heart disease has already shown itself. In an attempt to save the lives of those threatened in a first un-heralded attack of coronary thrombosis some hospitals have already installed intensive care units with automatic monitoring of heart rhythm and blood pressure and with day and night nursing care. Excellent as these are, their value has been questioned on the grounds that the urgent care should be available immediately and on the spot where the patient has been taken ill, for many do not survive the journey to hospital. This is valid criticism and should result in the formation of special medical emergency teams to deal with such cases before there is any question of their removal to hospital.

There are some forecasts which suggest that the rising curve of this disease is not likely to be halted since the stress of modern urban life is likely to increase rather than diminish. The concomitant antidotes – rich food, alcohol, tobacco, lack of physical effort and vigorous exercise – produce obesity and increased blood pressure as the arteries are narrowed by the layers of fat in their walls. When a thrombus (or blood clot) is caught in them to form a plug the heart is starved of blood. Drugs to reduce blood pressure will contribute to avoiding this crisis, and others to reduce obesity and to lower the level of cholesterol in the blood will also help. Preventive mass screening will produce a clearer picture of those at risk so that precautionary measures may be taken, and if a coronary attack does occur the patient will already be informed of what he should do until medical aid arrives. The value of such preventive action is underlined by the fact that coronary disease is extending its threshold of incidence to younger age groups and medical examination of army recruits in the United States has revealed premonitory symptoms in young men of twenty-five.

If, by all these methods, the number of fatal attacks is reduced, then the health of those who survive is likely to be greatly improved by surgical intervention. New coronary arteries supplied by venous homografts will help many, and where the heart has been damaged so that its action becomes dangerously irregular the cardiac pacemaker will restore it to normal rhythms. A new type of nuclear-powered pacemaker, designed to work for ten years without replacement, is already in use, and the implantation of a complete artificial heart is a practical possibility. Transplants of the whole lung as well as of the heart and other organs and vessels will become routine and will extend to those joints such as the knee where artificial replacements are likely to be unsatisfactory. Developments in surgery and anaesthetics generally, with automatic monitoring of post-operative patients, will greatly reduce the risks of major surgery. A further contribution to this end will be made by the widespread use of a prefabricated operating theatre, with all its ancillary rooms and services functionally designed, that can be erected within existing and obsolescent hospitals and so completely obviate the risks of infection that are inevitable in performing surgery in an environment that can never be completely controlled. Such a unit will have the further advantage that it can be frequently redesigned and replaced to meet new and unpredictable needs as surgery advances without structural alterations to the hospital building.

Although many infectious diseases are now satisfactorily controlled and others will certainly be brought under control by the use of new vaccines, the problems of infection will remain with us as more and more of the causative organisms become resistant to the present antibiotics. However, new antibiotics and new synthetic compounds will be found and these will include effective anti-viral agents. With growing knowledge of the way in which viruses affect cell metabolism it seems likely that new drugs will be highly specific in their action on certain viruses. The control of influenza will be more effective as the present vaccines are improved and as typing of the particular virus responsible is speeded up. But the control of the common cold is still likely to evade us, although more effective treatment of those affected will greatly shorten its course and minimize the risk of concurrent infections. Greater vigilance in enforcing present clean food legislation should make outbreaks of food poisoning more rare than they are now. The changing social habits and the increasing prosperity which encourages more and more people to eat in public restaurants will make this more necessary than ever.

The progress in immunochemistry, to which reference has already been made, will benefit research into the allergic disorders and their treatment as well as such diseases as rheumatoid arthritis, but the greatest progress is likely to be made in finding new drugs for mental illness. Already responsible for a major proportion of the demands for medical care, mental diseases are likely to increase steadily as the pace of social change increases. Many of the younger generation today, especially in the affluent societies, have experimented with drugs with more or less harmful effects. Addiction is not likely to diminish and will probably increase as new ways of life push more and more people to the edge of breakdown. Research is already going on to find new and safe drugs to deal with stress and as these prove themselves it is probable that their use will become socially acceptable.

This brief survey of probable trends in the prevention and treatment of disease makes it clear that medical and biological research will continue to demand a major effort, both in finance and manpower, if present possibilities are to be brought to fruition. Its task will never end for what we are asking of it is support in maintaining a balance between man and an ever-changing environment which becomes increasingly artificial and man-made. However successful the research may be, its beneficial application depends on social organization. Even in the United States today we are told that not everybody who is ill receives the best and most effective treatment to restore him to health, and how much more common must this situation be in many of the developing countries.

To counteract present economic trends, where we see rich countries becoming richer and poor countries poorer, more financial aid will have to be given the developing countries for their medical and welfare services. Just as the rich had to pay for the installation of pure water supplies and efficient sanitation for the poor in the industrial towns of the nine-teenth century, and with the same motives – that is to protect themselves and their children from the effects of epidemics that could begin there – so the rich countries will need to ensure that the principles of preventive medicine are every-where followed. The powerful international corporations with capital invested in the developing countries and with a growing need for a healthy and educated labour force to man their plants there will also contribute towards a levelling up of health standards throughout those countries. Some of the most widespread parasitic diseases there – malaria, schistoso-miasis and filariasis – can already be effectively controlled if the known preventive measures are employed. A gradual indoctrination of practitioners of native medicine among the vast populations of India and China with some of the basic principles of modern scientific medicine will make their work much more effective and help to solve the problem of providing basic medical care to people in rural areas. Peripatetic health teams and clinics will reinforce their efforts and help to counteract the over-centralization of medical care in large urban hospitals with scientifically trained doctors. The Soviet Union will certainly take an increasing share in supplying medical and welfare advisers to some developing countries, and their own urban model, with basic medical aid available in every large tenement block, together with their own variety of simple but effective health education, are likely to prove of value.

Nearer home, in our own National Health Service, measures of decentralization already begun with the establishment of the Area Boards will develop further. The completion of the Hospitals Building Plan will transform the hospital situation, but the new large district hospitals will be able to keep to their purpose of dealing with acute and serious emergencies more effectively as the local health centres develop and take their share of the burden of trivial recurrent ailments and much of the simple diagnosis and treatment which at present has to be carried by the outpatients' clinics. As new hospitals become available some of the old will be reorganized to become special hospitals for the aged and chronic sick, but in general the number of special hospitals, which are a physical outcome of nineteenth-century specialism, will be drastically reduced, for the new hospitals will have departments covering most of the medical specialties.

Highly trained medical manpower will continue in short supply, despite the recent increase in the number of those in training. Like all trained manpower, young doctors are learning to use their bargaining power and this will be used to increase job satisfaction and working conditions in hospitals.

As a result the present number of junior doctors on the establishment of hospitals will be doubled so that the work load may be reduced to reasonable proportions and study time be regularly taken. The folly of expecting any doctor to keep up to date in his knowledge without frequent periods of study leave will at last be appreciated and the organization of this will require yet more doctors to act as locums for those on study leave. The development of an integrated occupational medicine service will make a further demand on medical personnel, both doctors and nurses. This overdue reform would save the country hundreds of millions of pounds each year and more than pay for itself. Finally, as conditions improve and greater opportunities open up in their own countries, many of the young foreign doctors (now numbering more than 6,000) whose assistance keeps the hospital service from foundering will return home, either voluntarily or under pressure from their governments. Added to the number of young British doctors who leave to work abroad, this is likely to leave a considerable shortage which will take time and money to make good.

The effect of all this on the medical profession will be to produce further crises. Now that the financial prospects in general practice have been considerably improved, the incentive for young graduates to enter the long and arduous training necessary for hospital consultants is correspondingly less, and working conditions in the health centres, where doctors can really get to know their patients and their families, will add to the attraction of general practice. Old professional attitudes, with the specialist consultant at the top of a pyramid, will change drastically, but may be strong enough to raise another storm when, as it inevitably will, the proposal for a full-time salaried medical service is again brought forward. Another by no means distant prospect is a plan to introduce a medical auxiliary who will take some of the burden of routine medical care off the fully trained doctors. In the United States, where practically every doctor is some kind of specialist (a position which we shall certainly reach here) this is already a practical proposition. The kind of aide they intend to produce is a medical technician who can benefit from a special one year's 'crash course' which will train him to carry out simple diagnosis well enough to refer doubtful cases to a higher authority, to use the standard medical instruments and equipment, to prescribe standard medicaments and perform routine dressings. After these have been in action for a few years their work will be evaluated and is likely to be taken as an example to be followed elsewhere.

Advances in the social sciences will certainly have a great effect upon medicine. A great deal of research is already being carried out in the medical field by sociologists and much of it is proving effective in influencing the administrative policy of medical care. Investigations of the working of the health service at regional and local level will reveal anomalies and inadequacies at present buried in a mass of national statistics. Local involvement in medical care – something more than occasional protests at the closing of a local hospital – will again be as strong as it was in the days of the old voluntary hospitals. The new medico-social team responsible for local health and welfare services will need all the voluntary help it can get and the suggestion has been made that the idealism of the young might be usefully expressed in a year's compulsory national service in this field before they begin their university studies or take up full employment. As an exercise in health education alone, apart from the social benefits likely to develop from such a plan, it is worthy of serious consideration.

Whatever changes might be made in the financial basis of the health service – and wherever the money comes from the total must be increased – fears that it might be abandoned are groundless, for no responsible government could entertain such an idea when every other developed country which has not such a service already is moving towards it. Within the next decade, as the American Medical Association's reaction to the Carnegie Report indicates, the opposition there to federally based medical and welfare services is rapidly weakening and we are likely to see Medicare extended to cover all United States citizens whose income is below a certain level. Experimental pilot schemes of community medical care are already in operation with the aid of federal funds and these are likely to be expanded.

As all countries approach a certain common standard the interavailability of medical care will certainly be made far more general than it is today. The phenomenal growth of tourism during the past twenty-five years, when it has become the major earner of foreign currency for some countries, and its increasing growth in the coming decades will prove a major factor in bringing this about. These temporary migrations of millions of people, together with the rapid dissemination of information through the mass media will create a public opinion everywhere that is critical and demanding with relation to medical care and many other aspects of society. Pressure will grow upon governments to guard against the deterioration of the human environment upon purely economic grounds. It is useless to spend thousands of millions of pounds upon treating the sick if the quality of their life is to be continually devalued. Noise, traffic, air pollution, water pollution and overcrowding make life in any modern city a strain which erodes the resistance of the individual to disease.

Improved educational standards, not in Britain alone but throughout the world, will alert people to these dangers and many more specific issues of health and environment are likely to be the subject of organized protest and agitation. This is what democracy means, and an educated democracy will provide an electoral which is far more critical of all government action – or inaction – than it has ever been in the past. There is an element of idealism in all communal action that affects health, for the healthy man or woman does not worry about illness or think much about it. A breadwinner takes due care for his family, and a responsible citizen is prepared to see his money spent collectively to aid the sick and the needy who are less fortunate than himself. But he may be rightly critical of the organization of this aid and join with others to secure its improvement.

As certain minimum standards of medical care and welfare are achieved for the peoples of the developed countries many topics which are now great domestic issues will no longer attract interest and this element of idealism will be more generously extended to countries less fortunate. The very desirable spirit of adventure and restlessness characteristic of youth will find an outlet in voluntary youth service in these countries on a much greater scale than anything that has been attempted so far. As the people of Europe draw closer together in social and political union the continent which has had such a large part in creating our modern civilization will again assume its rightful importance in the world as a centre of stability and a source of new ideas and techniques in many of the fields we have been discussing. Their co-operation and aid will be of great value in solving many of the problems of the African countries.

If these observations seem to be straying rather far afield from the central theme of this book they follow necessarily from the role which medicine has to fill in a modern integrated society. It may serve and advise and teach but cannot dictate without altering the quality of life in ways that could be undesirable. Although, as we are told in Ecclesiasticus, 'Health is the most precious possession a man has. Health and

Bibliography

THE books listed below are arranged according to the chapters to which they are chiefly relevant. Inevitably there is some overlapping, and where this occurs the title is given only in the earliest chapter. Statistics are taken from the Annual Reports of the Department of Health and Social Security.

Chapter 1

ABSE, D. (1967) *Medicine on Trial*, Aldus Books, London.

CARTWRIGHT, A. (1967) *Patients and their Doctors*, Routledge & Kegan Paul, London.

Department of Health and Social Security (1970) *On the State of the Public Health*. The annual report of the Chief Medical Officer for the year 1969. H.M. Stationery Office, London.

GALDSTON, IAGO (1965) *Medicine in Transition*, University of Chicago Press, Chicago and London.

GLATT, M. M., *and others* (1967) *The Drug Scene in Great Britain*, Edward Arnold, London.

McKEOWN, T. (1965) *Medicine in Modern Society*, Allen & Unwin, London.

NORTON, ALAN (1969) *The New Dimensions of Medicine*, Hodder & Stoughton, London.

PAPPWORTH, M. H. (1967) *Human Guinea Pigs*, Routledge & Kegan Paul, London.

PINKER, R. (1966) *English Hospital Statistics, 1861–1938*, Heinemann, London.

POYNTER, F. N. L. *ed.* (1969) *Medicine and Culture*, Wellcome Institute of the History of Medicine, London.

SIMPSON, J., *and others* (1968) *Custom and Practice in Medical Care*, Oxford University Press, London.

STEVENS, R. (1966) *Medical Practice in Modern England*, Yale University Press, New Haven, Conn. and London.

TALAHAY, P. (1964) *Drugs in Our Society*, Johns Hopkins Press, Baltimore, Md. and Oxford University Press, London.

TITMUSS, R. M. (1971) *The Gift Relationship*, Allen & Unwin, London. This comprehensive study of the various methods employed in obtaining and supplying blood for transfusion services developed from Professor Titmuss's contribution to the symposium on 'Medicine and Culture'. See POYNTER (1969).

TOWNSEND, P. and WEDDERBURN, D. (1965) *The Aged in the Welfare State*, G. Bell, London.

WHITELEY, C. H. and WHITELEY, W. M. (1964) *The Permissive Morality*, Methuen, London.

Chapter 2

BELLERS, JOHN (1714) *An Essay towards the Improvement of Physick*, J. Sowle for J. Morphew, London.

HOBSON, W. (1963) *World Health and History*, Wright, Bristol.

JORDAN, W. K. (1960) *The Charities of London 1480–1660*, Allen & Unwin, London.

SHREWSBURY, J. F. D. (1970) *A History of the Bubonic Plague in England*, Cambridge University Press.

SIGERIST, H. E. (1944) *Civilization and Disease*, Cornell University Press, Ithaca, N.Y.

ZIEGLER, P. (1969) *The Black Death*, Collins, London.

ZINSSER, H. (1935) *Rats, Lice and History*, Boston, Mass., Little, Brown.

Chapter 3

CONNELL, A. M. and LINDEBOOM, G. A. eds. (1966) *The Christian Physician in the Advance of the Science and Practice of Medicine*, A. J. Oranje, The Hague. (Proceedings of the Second International Congress of Christian Physicians, Oxford, 11–15 July 1966.)

Contact: A quarterly journal whose aim is to promote a better understanding in the field of religion and medicine. Mowbrays, London.

EDMUNDS, V. and SCORER, C. G. (1958) *Ideals in Medicine*, Tyndale Press, London.

In the Service of Medicine: The Journal of the Christian Medical Fellowship (quarterly – No. 64 appeared in January 1971), C.M.F., London.

Chapter 4

GELFAND, M. (1968) *Philosophy and Ethics of Medicine*, Livingstone, Edinburgh.

LEDERMANN, E. K. (1970) *Philosophy and Medicine*, Tavistock Publications, London.

MEDAWAR, P. B. (1969) *Induction and Intuition in Scientific Thought*, Methuen, London.

TROTTER, W. (1941) *Collected Papers*, Oxford University Press, London.

Chapter 5

DOWNING, A. B. (1969) *Euthanasia and the Right to Die*, Peter Owen, London.

EBLING, F. J. (1969) *ed.*, *Biology and Ethics*, Academic Press, London and New York.

HINDELL, K. and SIMMS, M. (1971) *Abortion Law Reformed*, Peter Owen, London.
(N.B. This book was published in February 1971, too late to be consulted in the preparation of this volume.)

PICKENS, D. K. (1968) *Eugenics and the Progressives*, Vanderbilt University Press, Nashville, Tennessee.

STEVAS, N. St J. (1961) *Life, Death and the Law*, Eyre & Spottis-woode, London.

WILLIAMS, G. (1958) *The Sanctity of Life and the Criminal Law*, Faber & Faber, London.

WOLSTENHOLME, G. E. W. and O'CONNOR, M. *eds.*, *Ethics in Medical Progress*, Churchill, London.

Chapter 6

NEWMAN, C. (1957) *The Evolution of Medical Education in the Nineteenth Century*, Oxford University Press, London.

O'MALLEY, C. D. ed. (1970) *The History of Medical Education:* An International Symposium, University of California Press, Berkeley.

PICKERING, SIR G. (1967) *The Challenge to Education* (New Thinker's Library), Watts, London.

POYNTER, E. N. L. ed. (1966) *The Evolution of Medical Education in Britain*, Pitman Medical Publishing Co., London.

Report of the Royal Commission on Medical Education (Chairman, Lord Todd) (1968), H.M. Stationery Office, London.

Chapter 7

AYERS, G. M. (1971) *England's First State Hospitals 1867–1930* Wellcome Institute of the History of Medicine, London.

BEVERIDGE, LORD (1942) *Social Insurance and Allied Services* (Cmd. 6404), H.M. Stationery Office, London.

BRAND, J. L. (1965) *Doctors and the State*, Johns Hopkins Press, Baltimore, Md.

CLARK, C. (1967) *Population Growth and Land Use*, Macmillan, London.

ECKSTEIN, H. (1958) *The English Health Service*, Harvard University Press, Cambridge, Mass.

HODGKINSON, RUTH G. (1967) *The Origins of the National Health Service*, Wellcome Institute of the History of Medicine, London.

JEWKES, J. and JEWKES, S. (1961) *The Genesis of the British National Health Service*, Blackwell, Oxford.

JONES, K. (1960) *Mental Health and Social Policy, 1845–1959*, Routledge & Kegan Paul, London.

POWELL, ENOCH (1966) *A New Look at Medicine and Politics*, Pitman Medical Publishing Co. Ltd., London.

TITMUSS, R. M. (1958) *Essays on the Welfare State*, Allen & Unwin, London.

WOOTON, B. (1959) *Social Science and Social Policy*, Allen & Unwin, London.

Chapter 8

ABEL-SMITH, B. (1967) *An International Study of Health Expenditure*, W.H.O., Geneva.

BOTHWELL, P. W. (1965) *A New Look at Preventive Medicine*, Pitman Medical Publishing Co., London.

British Medical Association (1970) *Health Services Financing*. A report commissioned in 1967 by the B.M.A. and carried out by an Advisory Panel under the Chairmanship of Dr Ivor M. Jones, B.M.A., London.

GINZBERG, E. and OSTOW, M. (1969) *Men, Money, and Medicine*, Columbia University Press, New York, and London.

OFFICE OF HEALTH ECONOMICS (1962 onwards), *Publications*. More than 40 separate booklets containing condensed information on the cost of medical care, hospitals, drugs, etc.

TITMUSS, R. M. (1943) *Birth, Poverty, and Wealth. A Study of Infant Mortality*. Hamish Hamilton Medical Books, London.

Chapter 9

DUBOS, R. (1961) *The Dreams of Reason. Science and Utopias*, Columbia University Press, New York and London. (Especially Chapter 4 on 'Medical Utopias'.)

OFFICE OF HEALTH ECONOMICS (1969) *Medicines in the 1990s: a Technological Forecast*. O.H.E., London.

PAYNE, L. C. (1966) *An Introduction to Medical Automation*, Pitman Medical Publishing Co., London.

TAVERNER, D. (1968) *The Impending Medical Revolution*, Hodder & Stoughton, London.

Index

More about Penguins
and Pelicans

Penguinews, which appears every month, contains details of all the new books issued by Penguins as they are published. From time to time it is supplemented by *Penguins in Print*, which is a complete list of all available books published by Penguins. (There are well over four thousand of these.)

A specimen copy of *Penguinews* will be sent to you free on request, and you can become a subscriber for the price of the postage. For a year's issues (including the complete lists) please send 30p if you live in the United Kingdom, or 60p if you live elsewhere. Just write to Dept EP, Penguin Books Ltd, Harmondsworth, Middlesex, enclosing a cheque or postal order, and your name will be added to the mailing list.

Note: *Penguinews* and *Penguins in Print* are not available in the U.S.A. or Canada

The Penguin Medical Encyclopedia

PETER WINGATE

Hippocrates asserted, over two thousand years ago, that a doctor must teach his patients to care for their own health. Until recently, however, most doctors have preferred to believe that patients can know too much.

This encyclopedia is deliberately addressed to patients and not to the medical profession, though nurses may well find it invaluable. At the same time Dr Wingate (who regularly broadcasts on medical topics) is emphatic that it is not a 'Home Doctor' or do-it-yourself medical manual.

In hundreds of entries, running from *abdomen* to *zymosis*, he covers anatomy and the diseases of body and mind; drugs and surgery; the history, institutions and vocabulary of the profession; and many other aspects of medicine and psychology. In the course of these Dr Wingate clearly explains the principles involved in the diagnosis and treatment of a thousand and one illnesses from the inconvenience of baldness to the rigours of cancer.

Not for sale in the U.S.A. or Canada

Man, Medicine, and Environment
RENÉ DUBOS

In this book Dr Dubos, an editor of the *Journal of Experimental Medicine*, examines the environmental forces affecting the history of social groups from the precursors of *homo sapiens* to man today. Considering characteristics unique to humanity, he states that 'Man can function well only when his external environment is in tune with the needs he has inherited from his evolutionary, experiential and social past, and with his aspirations for the future.' As man acquires much of his personality through responses to environment, Dr Dubos discusses the complex interrelations that govern life today, and the effects of environment on the health of primitive and modern man. In non-technical language he surveys the control of life, biomedical philosophies and the possibilities of a science of man. Precisely because they are concerned with various aspects of humanity, Dr Dubos believes that 'the biomedical sciences in their highest form are potentially the richest expression of science'.

Not for sale in the U.S.A. or Canada